EDUCATION IN A COMPETITIVE AND GLOBALIZING WORLD

HEALTH PROMOTION IN SCHOOL

THEORY, PRACTICE AND CLINICAL IMPLICATIONS

EDUCATION IN A COMPETITIVE AND GLOBALIZING WORLD

Additional books in this series can be found on Nova's website under the Series tab.

Additional e-books in this series can be found on Nova's website under the e-book tab.

EDUCATION IN A COMPETITIVE AND GLOBALIZING WORLD

HEALTH PROMOTION IN SCHOOL

THEORY, PRACTICE AND CLINICAL IMPLICATIONS

ANTONIO IUDICI, M.D.

nova publishers
New York

NOTICE TO THE READER

Library of Congress Cataloging-in-Publication Data

ISBN: 978-1-63117-705-7

Published by Nova Science Publishers, Inc. † New York

CONTENTS

ABSTRACT

In addition to the role of educating the citizens of the future, schools today respond to other social needs, especially in promoting health. A school is a key place to impact the thinking of young people through various social situations, such as teachers and educators dealing with issues that may not be faced within the family (e.g. knowledge of sexually transmitted diseases); treating certain themes through peer group settings (for example, learning to discuss topics of interest with someone of the same age in the presence of an adult guide); facilitating the understanding of different cultural norms (for example, developing knowledge of certain social rules or offenses for foreign students); and finally, allowing young people to interpret the promotion of health as a collective responsibility that has multiple steps.

Schools have increasingly needed the help of professionals from the educational and psychological fields. Examples of this would be the requests for specialist assistance in dealing with "difficult" or "unmanageable" children, and courses in school that teach tobacco or drugs prevention, anti-bullying, sex education, etc. In fact, all you need to ensure proper health promotion in schools is a synergetic combination of the issues of health and education. Yet, work in schools on health issues is not always easy, especially in terms of certain issues: finding a common line among experts and teachers is difficult; time to work together on projects is limited; often there is no project evaluation; external professionals have trouble finding time while school is in session to come to a school; principals and teachers are not willing to deal with health issues; there is a lack of cooperation on the part of the students' parents; the school's program and the national health plan are not well regulated; and students tend to listen passively and are unwilling to be directly involved. Therefore, a significant social responsibility for health promotion is placed on schools without adequate support being available to them. Schools should be provided with the resources and educational skills necessary for them to address the issues that society requires them to deal with. This work seeks to create a link between health promotion and schools, to describe the various theoretical approaches to health promotion currently existing world-wide, to perform a historical analysis of some issues that affect health at school (smoking, bullying, deviance, intercultural issues etc.), and to present some operative interventions for the benefit of school leaders, teachers, parents, educators, and psychologists.

Keywords: Health promotion, School education, School psychology, Clinical, Social science, Tobacco, Deviance, Bullying, Intercultural

PREFACE

Everywhere in the world, school, being one of the most important institutional landmarks, has always represented a society. Since states first decided to establish places for children's education, a school has been a place for learning, for knowledge for education, and for the formation of the young citizenry. Its role in hosting children during their growth path makes the school a unique place in which to interact with new generations. After all, school is a crossroads of ways and ideas through which children and parents relate with the institutions.

For these reasons, the school is asked to respond to social needs such as educating the community, raising a responsible citizenry, and developing certain social skills. With international regulations, schools should develop useful skills for adequate social integration, promoting the full realization of the society itself (WHO, UN, WTO, OECD).

However, there are some obstacles to this realization. For example, school has always been considered the main venue in which knowledge is exclusively transmitted. Thanks to an interactive educational system that tends to be one-sided, school has been identified primarily with the curricular materials included in it. This has resulted in the inability of schools to take external initiatives with the endorsement of their ministries. External agencies have their own agenda when they are called to contribute to educational services or to psychosocial services. They deal with merely informative content, often medicalizing the culture of health to which they were appointed. Initiatives against tobacco or drug abuse have resulted in behavioral prescriptions or informative lists of the effects of the substances, as well as informative activities designed to teach children how to avoid sexually transmitted diseases and to understand the importance of contraceptive methods. Following the application of the medical model, these interventions were labeled "prevention" and not "health promotion". The trends described have created considerable confusion about the functions assigned to the school. On one hand, a school is a cultural place in which many social skills are developed; on the other, it is a place where there is a fragmented transmission of knowledge. In parallel, there has been a difference in the understanding of students. In the first case they are considered active subjects who change their school participation based on various social changes; on the other hand they are considered passive users in the same way that containers are used to store objects. The confusion explained above is present in the everyday lives of the students, teachers, parents, etc. From this, a profound de-legitimization of the entire school institution results with a growing increase in school drop-outs and talks aimed at discrediting it. In spite of everything, the international community and school standards have agreed that school is a place for the formation of the citizenry, and a place to develop skills, especially psychosocial skills. You can see there is a perfect relationship between school and health. The aim of the school is to help students to live a better life. The participation of the citizen depends on how we are trained. Unlike studying and knowing the way in which students can construct situations, well-being can facilitate the acquisition of what the school offers in terms of both cultural and relational notions. We are interested in strengthening the relationship between school and health promotion. The main aim of this book is to offer all people who work in schools (teachers, project managers of health promotion, educators, psychologists, social workers) the conceptual and normative references (also in terms of history) and some indications of a method to create a scientifically founded idea of health promotion.

The text consists of two parts: the first presents how health and disease were understood historically and describes the theories, approaches, and scientific paradigms that have theorized the concept of health.

The second part describes the general assumptions of health promotion in school and some topics that have become particularly difficult to manage in the last decade, inside the school and involving both the school and health. In relation to these issues, we describe the main approaches to the topic and its critical issues, and we offer some methodological guidance. These interventions in schools must be considered according to the specific context and the resources present. This book is devoted to exposing some macro intervention criteria as current practise does not respond to the need for school personnel to develop their own skills, or "the ability to think".

Of course, this book does not intend to exhaust all that can be said about the actions of health promotion in school, but it represents an attempt to connect the two areas, school and health, which have been unjustifiably kept at a distance for years - even in the face of the scarcity of contributions to literature and the noticeable absence of scientific references that would lay them in comparison.

ACKNOWLEDGEMENTS

I would like to thank Dr. Valeria Gherardini for collaboration on Chapter 2, Dr. Antonello Andrea for collaboration on Chapter 4, Dr. Nicolò De Franceschi for collaboration on Chapter 6, Dr. Guido Pasquale for collaboration on Chapter 7, and Professor Elena Faccio for the stimuli and encouragement in the preparation of this work.

About the Author

Antonio Iudici, M.D., PsyS, psychotherapist, is a professor of the Department of Philosophy, Education, Sociology and Applied Psychology (FISPPA) of the University of Padova (Italy). Dr. Iudici is a researcher associate at the Institute of Psychology and Psychotherapy of Padova.

PART ONE

Chapter 1

HEALTH PROMOTION: HISTORY OF THE CONCEPT AND REFERENCE STANDARDS

1. INTRODUCTION

The concept of health is important not only for the content that it offers to the community, but also because it helps to create new services and new disciplinary figures. Today, the average citizen deals with a great number of different disciplines and operators that belong to different institutions. Health promotion does not have a specific discipline, but its realization is favored by psychology, the educational sciences, medicine, the social sciences, and the decisions of administrators and politicians.

Health promotion is primarily a cultural and institutional community practice because of its complexity and multiplicity.

Similarly, the objectives pursued are not geared exclusively to the modification of individual behavior, but rather to promoting schemes and ways of reasoning from which it generates the same behavior in a community. Although the issue of health has been discussed in different historical periods, with different meanings and manifestations, only in the 1980s and 1990s did it become an international and institutional formalization. We can see that this recent formalization has represented a key moment for the organization of social and health services, resulting in some significant changes in cultural policies and especially organizational services.

2. History of the Concept

The first studies we have about health came from the Greeks in the form of the studies of Hippocrates (470-377 B.C.), who is considered the father of medicine. He considered good health to be the harmonious balance of an organism. In the absence of such a balance, there would be illness. Hippocrates extended this concept to other areas such as the conditions of life and all environments. Hippocrates approached some of our current health dietetics. "Ancient *diaita* has to do with the life of man in its totality. La *diaita* uses *physis*, growing and naturally, getting the *nomos*, the right size and rule of the culture of a governed life. This isn't possible without *paideia*, without instruction and guide, without *arete,* the virtue, and *sophrosyne,* the discernment, without education in the organic environment that the ancients called cosmos, the wonderful order of a harmonious universe" [1]. For many centuries, diseases were considered an imbalance of bodily elements and these in turn were associated with an imbalance of the soul. Centuries earlier, medicine had been associated with religion, but Hippocrates succeeded in separating medicine from religion.

In the medieval period, the term "health" was seen in a spiritual way, and often seen as a part of nature. It was considered the opposite of disease. A person's "well-being" or healthy life, as opposed to disease, was compared with a complex relationship between God, man and nature. Man is seen to be independent from God; therefore, accidents and illness are considered the consequences of rebellion or denial of God [2]. Man has become *homo rebellis* and now has to carry his inner conflict. In this struggle, illness is the problematic expression of disease, enclosed in the key concept of black bile melancholia [3]. Today the notion of the protection of the spirit prevailing on the care of the sick, being the most important existential function of healing [4], has been forgotten. In that period, it was believed that illness was the punishment of God which is why people asked for intercession to some specific saints: Saint Biagio was known as the protector of the throat, Saint Appollonia for teeth, Saint Lorenzo for the back, Saint Bernardino for the lungs, and Saint Erasmus for the abdomen. Only in the late medieval period did Saint Isidore of Seville in his etymologies say that medicine was not a part of art. In this way medicine was approached according to the philosophy that if philosophy is behind the care of the human spirit then we find ourselves very far from how medicine and philosophy were described [5].

It is useful to realize that concepts of both health and illness were different but very common. Healthy living was not a specified discipline until it was considered a liberal art. The conceptions of health and illness were not defined topics for a long time — not until almost the end of the 1700s. Diseases like malaria, cholera smallpox, typhoid fever and tuberculosis were allocated from time to time to non-medical pathology. Jews, for example, were accused of intentionally spreading the plague. The first hospital was based on the charitable support of volunteers, not on the principles of medical healing. This was when mendicant orders were founded (Dominicans and Franciscans) and military orders of chivalry created structures in which there was no distinction between the sick, pilgrims, and beggars. Only around 1500 did they start to postulate that illness was something from nature and not from God. This can be seen in *De contagione et contagiosis* by Girolamo Fracastoro (1478-1553), which is based on the assumption that small living particles called *seminarie* were first spread by direct contact with materials or the air. In many cases, pro-conservation officials, guards with specific powers, or permanent magistrates were entrusted with the task of controlling hygienic conditions.

In the 1700s, clinical institutions were introduced by overcoming the distance between universities and hospitals and for the first time doctors were paid [6].

States only assumed the exercise of care in the eighteenth and nineteenth centuries. The principles of secularism and the rationality of public administration sometimes came into conflict with ecclesiastical structures. In the 1800s some innovative methods were introduced, such as vaccination. This was the period in which chemistry and biology were used to intervene against illness. In this period illness became a public topic as Artelt [7] supported this organization, based on controlling the population, which was managed by internal ministers. You can find them all over the world.

Throughout the twentieth century, there then developed an exasperated technicality that led to the identification of the individual with only one "side" and "body," reducing the overall idea of the person. The culture of health as the absence of disease or disablement has meant that the majority of technological investments have been dedicated to reducing or eliminating disease or symptoms. But the definition of health must be expanded in a better way.

It is left to us to understand the relationship between illness and the environment, as well as to learn how to construct an effective and global well-being. Humans were so far from the idea that there is a relationship between man's illness and the improper use of the environment. However, this was the moment in which public health care systems begins to be established. Because of the idea that health is to be considered a human right, various ministries were especially established and organized from different international ministries, including the World Health Organization.

3. Reference Standards

The World Health Organization concerns itself with health issues. It was founded in 1946 and enforced in 1948 by the victors of the Second World War (China, France, Russia, the United Kingdom, and the United States) with 44 signatories. It replaced the League of Nations, which had been established after the First World War to guarantee peace and security. Today it has 194 members; its decision-making body is the World Health Assembly, comprising of representatives of each country's health administration (ministries of health). Its aim is to make sure every country attains a high level of health, as it claims in its founding statutes. After the WHO was founded, attention has been focused on the concept of health.

The term health has taken on a variety of meanings. These terms have defined more precisely the areas of intervention related to the constructs of disease and health. In fact, if the preceding era had been characterized by a focus on the concept of disease, after the creation of the WHO, organizations' focus gradually shifted to the concept of health.

- Constitution of the World Health Organization in 1948.

  According to the WHO in 1948, "Health is a state of complete physical and mental and social well-being, not just the absence of illness or disablement. To enjoy high standards of health is one of the fundamental rights of every human being without health distinction, race, religion, political beliefs etc. The health of all is important for the achievement of peace, and security is dependent on the wider co-operation of individuals and states. The state's efforts in health promotion and protection are useful to all, while unequal development in promoting health can cause problems. For in this case all conditions, such as social status, education, occupation, household income, may affect health in negative or in positive ways" [8].
- Declaration of Alma-Ata in 1978.

  The International Conference on Primary Health Care met in Alma-Ata on September 12, 1978. During the conference the need for urgent action by all governments, health and development workers, and the world community to protect and promote the health of all the people of the world was expressed. The Conference strongly reaffirmed that health, which was defined as a state of complete physical, mental, and social well-being, and not merely the absence of disease or infirmity, is a fundamental human right and that the attainment of the highest possible level of health is an important world-wide social goal. The realization of this requires the action of many other social and economic sectors in addition to the health sector [9].

The conference at Alma-Ata declared that health is a fundamental right of every human being. The statement is particularly important as it explicitly names, for the first time, the target of reference, which is to achieve the highest possible level of health for the whole world.

- Ottawa Charter in 1986.

This document speaks about health intervention, stating that health promotion is "the process of enabling people to increase their control over and to improve their health. To reach a state of complete physical, mental, and social well-being, an individual or group must be able to identify aspirations, to satisfy needs, and to cope with the environment. Therefore, health is seen as a resource for everyday life, not the objective of living. Health is a positive concept emphasizing social and personal resources, as well as physical capabilities. Health promotion is not just the responsibility of the health sector, but goes beyond healthy life-styles to well-being" [10].

The Charter of Ottawa calls attention to the responsibility of all sectors, inviting them to full awareness of the health consequences of their decisions. Health is a concept which needs to be promoted and to do so you need to create reasonable public policies, a good environment, health services, and anything else that can help to improve health education, such as culture, transportation, agriculture, tourism etc.

- Bangkok Charter for Health Promotion in a Globalized World in 2005.

The Bangkok Charter identifies the actions, commitments, and pledges required to address the determinants of health in a globalized world through health promotion. The Bangkok Charter affirms that the policies and partnerships required to empower communities and to improve health and health equality should be at the center of global and national development. Health promotion has been defined by the

World Health Organization in 2005 as the process of enabling people to increase control over their health and its determinants, and thereby improve their overall health. It is a core function of public health and contributes to the work of tackling communicable and non-communicable diseases and other threats to health [11]. The primary means of health promotion occur through developing public health policy that addresses the prerequisites of health such as income, housing, food security, employment, and good-quality working conditions [12, 13, and 14].

To make further advances in implementing these strategies, all sectors must:

- Have advocates for health based on human rights and solidarity;
- Invest in sustainable policies, actions, and infrastructure that address determinants of health;
- Produce the capacity for policy development, leadership, health promotion practice, knowledge transfer and research, and health literacy;
- Legislate regulations that ensure a high level of protection from harm and enable equal opportunities for health and well-being; and
- Collaborate and build alliances with public, private, and international organizations to create sustainable actions.

4. From the Bio-Medical Model to the Bio-Psycho-Social Model

In reference to how the social sciences can use the standard references mentioned above, we can now highlight a few key points to design interventions in society and in schools.

Now, you will notice how health evolved from the medieval period to modern times. The constant reference to biological, psychological, and social dimensions makes it impossible to reduce health promotion to medical intervention. Yet, the interventions of health services have had, as a point of reference, a model - named biomedical - based on the healing of illness, which is understood as:

a) An alien entity from which the individual is affected;
b) An entity that must be studied, treated, and separated from the individual affected and preserved by subjective variables identified as a disorder to reduce or eliminate;
c) A condition experienced as egodystonic, the implication of which is the ideological belief that a person does not want to get sick or healed [15].

This setting has denied the psychological and social influences in determining the conditions that generate disease. The limit of this approach, recognized by international literature [16, 17, 18, 19, 20, 21, and 22], was not to consider how this influence could affect the disease, which has obviously always been postulated as being totally independent of the individual, both in its genesis and in its effect.

The new conceptualizations have not only extended the area of health as well as that of the body, but they have also rightfully included both psychological and social connections. These changes have disrupted many public health services around the world, which have been accustomed to acting exclusively on health aspects, but which are not ready to deal with other aspects, such as psychological issues.

From this comes the need to renovate the organization of hospital services in regard to the aspects described above, but this has been undertaken tardily by most countries of the world, especially those in which medicine is used to reduce fears and anxieties. This in turn has produced a need to renovate many practices and medical procedures based solely on the body.

The health of our bodies, while important, is not a compelling indicator of health. Preceding it in importance are the skills needed to improve the welfare of the individual to reduce the conditions that cause disease. The ability to find an environment with proper health conditions is psychosocial. In fact, the Ottawa Charter defined personal and social resources [10]. Furthermore, the acquisition and the development of these resources must be considered in light of the promotion of a greater consciousness of humanity, from which is deduced an "active" connotation of man, hoping for a change in the environment and social context in which he lives [23]. This is considered along with the epidemiological and demographic changes that characterize our time (i.e. aging, excessive eating habits, drug use, social distress, etc.).

Even new social phenomena, related and unrelated to bodily function, can be identified from different models. No longer limited to the sphere of sickness or absence of disease, these models blend biological, psychological, and social aspects of health.

The opposition to this cultural change is still great, especially in those areas of public health in which there are many economic interests. From an organizational point of view, the switch is opposed by procedures that always categorize according to the criterion of pathogenesis and by the salutogenic approach [19, 22, 24, and 25]. The latter relates to the ways in which health is generated, identifying the process. In this case, the researcher's focus is not solely on those infected with a disease, but on the ways in which people adopt habits that prevent disease [26]. This involves locating that healthy "sense of coherence" which Antonovsky [22, 24, 27, and 28] defines through three components: understandability, manageability, and significance. Understandability is the degree to which the bearer perceives events. Manageability is the degree to which a person can manage him or herself. Significance is the sense a person has for taking the challenges associated with life.

In general, understanding and studying the processes through which health is generated must empower all social disciplines in order for their epistemological, technical, and application contribution to be realized.

Although the references described above have broad implications for health promotion, there is no precise definition of what health is. Many critics consider the Ottawa Charter to be abstract and utopian in its pursuits. Many of the execution models suffer from conflicting conceptual hypotheses.

REFERENCES

[1] Jori, A. (1996). *Medicina e medici nell'antica Grecia. Saggio sul "Perì téchnes" ippocratico*. Bologna: Il Mulino editore.

[2] Osler, W. (1913). *The Evolution of Modern Medicine.* Yale University Press.

[3] Schipperges, H. (1988). *Il giardino della salute: la medicina nel medioevo.* Milano: Garzanti.

[4] Phillips, E.D. (1973), *Aspects of Greek Medicine*. New York: St. Martin's Press.

[5] Cosmacini G., Gaudenzi, G., Satolli R. (a cura di) (1996). *Dizionario di storia della salute.* Torino: G. Einaudi.

[6] Rossi, P. (1997). *La nascita della scienza moderna in Europa*. Roma-Bari: Laterza.

[7] Artelt, W. (1949). *Einfuhrung in die Medizinhistorik: Ihr Wesen, ihre Arbeitsweise und ihre Hilfsmittel*. Stuttgart: Enke.
[8] World Health Organization (1948). World Health Organization constitution. In *Basic documents*. Geneva: World Health Organization.
[9] World Health Organization (1978). *Declaration of Alma-Ata: International conference on primary health care, Alma-Ata, USSR, 6–12 September 1978*. Retrieved February 14, 2006, from http://www.who.int/hpr/NPH/docs/ declaration_almaata.pdf
[10] World Health Organization (1986). *The Ottawa charter*. Geneva: World Health Organization.
[11] Comitato Nazionale per la Bioetica (2001). *Orientamenti bioetici per l'equità nella salute*. Presidenza del Consiglio dei ministri Dipartimento per l'Informazione e l'Editoria.
[12] World Health Organization (2005). *The Bangkok Charter for Health Promotion in a Globalized World*. 6th Global Conference on Health Promotion. Available at: [Accessed: March 23, 2007].
[13] World Health Organization (2005). *Update of the Health Promotion Glossary*, unpublished observations. Geneva: World Health Organization.
[14] World Health Organization (2000). *Health Systems: Improving Performance*. The World Health Report 2000. Geneva: World Health Organization.
[15] Tartarotti, L. (2010). *Psicologia della salute: un'introduzione*. Milano: Franco Angeli.
[16] Foucault, M. (1969). *Nascita della clinica*. Torino: Einaudi.
[17] Ongaro Basaglia, F. (1982). *Salute/Malattia Le parole della medicina*. Torino: Einaudi.
[18] Braibanti, P. (2004). *Pensare salute: orizzonti e nodi critici della Psicologia della Salute*. Milano: Franco Angeli.
[19] Bertini, M. (2012). *Psicologia della Salute*. Roma: Raffaello Cortina.
[20] Zani B., & Cicognani E. (2000). *Psicologia della salute*. Bologna: Il Mulino.
[21] Eriksson, M., & Lindström, B. (2010). Bringing it all together: The salutogenic response to some of the most pertinent public health dilemmas. In: Morgan, A., Davies, M., Ziglio, E. (eds). *Health Assets in a Global Context. Theory, Methods, Action* (p 339-351). New York: Springer.
[22] Antonovsky, A. (1979). *Health, stress and coping*. Washington: Jossey-Bass.

[23] Bennett, P., & Murphy, S. (1997). *Psychology and health promotion, health psychologist series*. Buckingham: Open University Press Buckingham.

[24] Antonovsky, A. (1987). *Unravelling the mystery of health*. San Fransisco, Jossey-Bass

[25] Macdonald, J.J. (2005). *Environments for health*. London: Earthscan.

[26] Morgan, A., Davies, M., & Ziglio, E. (eds). *Health Assets in a Global Context. Theory, Methods, Action*. New York: Springer.

[27] Antonovsky A. (1993). The structure and properties of the sense of coherence scale. *Soc Sci Med;* 36, p. 725–33.

[28] Antonovsky A (1996). The salutogenic model as a theory to guide health promotion. *Health Promotion International*, 11(1), p. 11–18.

Chapter 2

Different Approaches to Health Promotion

1. Introduction

With the inclusion of psychological and social aspects in the definitions of health, we can see how health is connected with these different aspects. This new approach is called the bio-psycho-social model, which is unique for its various aspects mentioned in the biomedical model characteristics of the period before the OMS definition.

2. Psychological Theories

Increased openness regarding matters not limited to the medical field has produced psychological contributions to the development which have attempted to explain health behaviors, coming mainly from the field of Social Cognition.

1 - Health Belief Model

This approach stems from the need to understand the reasons for which people are not subjected to diagnostic evaluations to verify the presence or absence of a disease, in particular because of a physician's request. The authors [1] hypothesized, according to other studies [2, 3], the presence of psychological variables at the root of the decision not to undergo testing. They therefore formalized a model based on the belief that healthy behavior is mediated by: the perception of the severity (perceived severity), the perception of vulnerability (perceived susceptibility), the degree of advantages of behavior, understood as the product between the perceived benefits (perceived benefits) and the perceived costs (perceived barriers). The perception of severity refers to the degree of seriousness attributed to the disease or the potential damage and its consequences. The perception of vulnerability is understood as the degree to which one feels at risk of contracting the disease. The perceived benefits indicate those benefits that the person attributes to him/herself by changing his/her own behavior, while the perceived costs are the extent of the difficulties, barriers, or efforts that could lead to a modification of their behavior. This approach is primarily based on an assessment of cognitive processes that people could experience regarding a specific behavior on the health-illness continuum.

2 - Protection Motivation Theory

This approach is based on the idea that a healthy behavior is achievable through the construct of motivation to protect (protection motivation). This construct is theorized to be the result of two measurement processes, the perception of intensity (threat appraisal) and the perception of being able to implement protective responses (coping appraisal). This approach has been developed through studies that have taken place over a period of about 12 years by different authors [3, 4, 5]. The final processing of this approach defines motivation protection as consisting of the following sub-processes: the perceived severity, the perceived vulnerability, efficacy response, cost response, the rewards of maladaptive responses and self-efficacy.

The perceived severity indicates the self-perceived measure of seriousness of the disease. The perceived vulnerability refers to the extent to which we believe ourselves to be personally exposed to the disease. The self-efficacy response indicates the benefits received by individuals in changing their behavior with respect to the disease. The cost response is the measure of effort, labor and the consequences that we are willing to accept after acting for a change. The rewards of maladaptive responses refer to the advantages of not changing one's behavior. In clinical terms, the expression "secondary benefits" is often used and refers to the indirect benefits, especially for the maintenance of a non-healthy behavior (e.g. "eating gives me a feeling of relief", "drinking helps me to forget", or jeopardizing one's ankle by wearing high heels for the 'benefit' of appearing elegant). The self-efficacy process refers to the perception of self-efficacy in the establishment of the desired behaviors.

Some conceptualizations have also affected the studies of other authors, such as, for example, the work of Lazarus [7] and Bandura [8].

3 - Reasoned Action Theory

This approach comes from studies by Fishbein and Ajzen [9, 10]. The focal point of this approach is the relationship between attitude and behavior. The authors, Fishbein and Ajzen, focused on health protection behavior, and the attempt to implement desired behavior by changing attitude. This attempt is achieved by two processes: altering the individual's attitude toward the desired behavior and helping the individual to reject subjective social norms that guide his/her choices.

This attempt to change behavior is mediated by two additional micro-processes: altering the individual's beliefs about the behavior's consequences (behavior beliefs, beliefs about how our behavior will produce a result) and how the individual values the consequences of the behavior (evaluations of behavioral change outcomes, i.e. what value we attach to those consequences). Subjective norms that lead to a choice are in turn divided into normative beliefs (normative beliefs, the relationship between the changes we make and what others think of those changes) and the value placed on conformity (motivation to comply, the value attributed to others' interpretations of how we have changed).

Although this approach has been used extensively in various fields, social psychology has many times emphasized that attitude does not explain behavior and this relationship. The two are not significantly correlated [11, 12, 13, 14, 15, 16].

4 - Planned Behavior Theory

This approach is to be considered a development of *Reasoned Action Theory*. One of the two authors of this method, Icek Ajzen [17, 18], introduced in the previous model the construct of perceived control behavior, which refers to the perception of how to control the desired behavior, for example by highlighting the degree of difficulty or the ease of implementing action. Even the *Planned Behavior Theory* is based on the behavioral intention construct, i.e. on the intention to implement the desired behavior. This intention is mediated by three processes, of which the first two are identical to those of the approach of *Reasoned Action Theory*:

1) The intention toward the behavior is mediated by two additional micro-processes: the beliefs about the behavior consequences (behavior beliefs, beliefs about the results of the behavior) and consequences value (evaluations of behavioral outcome; namely, the value attached to those consequences);
2) Subjective norms that lead to a choice are divided into the normative beliefs (the relationship between our change and what others think of that change) and compliance attributed value (motivation to comply, the value attributed to how others interpret our change).
3) Perceived behavioral control, or the perception of being able to control the behavior that you want to change [19].
4) According to some studies [20, 21, 22], the introduction of this construct makes this approach more effective than the one defined by Fishbein and Ajzen.

5 - Health Action Process Approach

This approach was formalized by the German psychologist Schwartzer [23, 24] and is based on the idea that the adoption of health behaviors and the maintenance thereof are mediated by motivational and volitional constructs. The first two constructs refer to the intention formation, while the latter indicates the planning of the concrete. The intention is configured as a decision-making process that involves the perception of risk (defined with respect to perceived severity and perceived vulnerability) and outcome expectations (including social outcomes). From the perception of risk comes the process of defining the expectations of the outcome and, hence, the incentive to respond effectively (perception of self-efficacy) [25, 26]. The self-efficacy construct is also important for the strong-willed, as it is believed that a plan of action is constructed in relation to the abilities that a person attributes to him/herself. The self-efficacy construct could help to prefigure scenarios, restricting a person's ability to move through the trial-and-error method [27]. The next part is about the implementation phase and involves cognitive and behavioral aspects, specifically the action planning and control or strategies identification process to prevent schedule interruption.

6 - Trans-Theoretical Model of Behavior Change

DiClemente and Prohaska [28, 29] developed this approach, which is called the *integrated model*, as it brings together constructs that belong to several different theories. However, it can be used in a variety of different contexts, such as behavioral techniques, psychotherapy, mutual self-aid groups, and counseling. The model follows these constructs: stages of change, processes of change, decisional balance, and self-efficacy. The authors started from the assumption that their studies concerned the ineffectiveness of certain media prevention campaigns, which take for granted that the person to whom they are addressed has already decided to change. According to the authors, there are different levels of motivation to change. What characterizes this approach, unlike other models, is the difference in consequential stages. Each stage represents a specific level of motivation and at the base of that motivation there are different psychological processes that must be considered to change behavior. In fact, the model predicts different tasks and activities in which the subject will have to participate, depending on his or her mental state [30]. The model was created through the use of *ad hoc* instruments, mainly questionnaires. The idea that there are different levels of motivation has actually opened up new possibilities for action by meeting the need of many operators active in the healthcare sector. Until this idea was theorized, the change in behavior was thought of as an "all or nothing" activity [31]. This aspect and the ease of its application explain the success of this approach, applied especially to dieting, early diagnosis of disease, use of condoms, and so on [32, 33]. The stages are described as follows:

In the transtheoretical model, change is a "process involving progress through a series of stages":

- Precontemplation (Not Ready) - The subject is not motivated to implement changes and does not recognize his/her status as problematic. Consequently, he/she evades any discourse intended to cause changes in his/her actions.
- Contemplation (Getting Ready) - The subject begins to consider his/her condition as a problem and so considers the opportunity to make changes. However, at this stage, the relationship between the

change and those advantages in maintaining the situation as it is appear erratic, making the situation unstable.

- Preparation (Ready) - The subject has decided to make changes to his/her own situation as soon as he/she can. This is the change and assessment planning stage.
- Action - The subject brings about his/her decision, experiencing the effects of his/her changes. The subject also attempts to identify strategies to resist the possible consequences.
- Maintenance - The subject keeps the changes actively implemented with self-efficacy and responds to situations that can destabilize the changes obtained and the benefits associated with them.
- Termination - The subject has no temptations and is sure not to return to the advantages of the above conditions. He/she owns and applies coping strategies in relation to all risks.

In the 1983 version of the model, the Termination stage is not present. In the 1992 version of the model, Prochaska et al. [29, 31] showed Termination as the end of their "Spiral Model of the Stages of Change", rather than separating it.

The authors have also conceptualized the condition of "relapse", recycling, which consists in returning to earlier stages. However, this is not a true study [34].

7 - The Model of Mediating Variables in Health

This approach, defined by Rutter, Quine and Cheshman [35], is based on the construct of coping, which is understood as the way in which people face their own complex problems and endure them. The authors, starting from the aspect of health deficiencies that may have originated from some life events (such as marriage, social class, income, housing, employment), formalize the presence of two variables: the affective and the cognitive disposition. These variables are correlated with the construct "coping," which can affect variables and influence decisions. A dysfunction in the management of coping behaviors can lead to poor health choices, such as smoking, drinking, etc.

8 - Conner and Norman Model

The authors of this model identify five stages at the base of behavior change related to healthy behaviors. This approach attempts to focus on the link between emotional, and motivational components, and the act of switching from intentionality to action.

The first stage is defined as pre-reflective, in which the subject does not consider the possibility of changing his/her behavior. At this stage, only external stimuli can encourage other ideas, i.e. events that cause a reflection or a perceived danger. In the second stage, known as motivation and decision, the subject is motivated to act. This is mediated by outcome expectations, social influences, and personal experiences.

The third stage, called planning, involves an action plan developed by the subject and the processes of construction for the subject's personality to mediate it.

The fourth and fifth stages, called action and maintenance, involve the monitoring and control of the subject's own behavior.

Transverse to these stages is the construct of self-efficacy which facilitates the passage from one stage to another [36].

9 - The Anticipatory Emotion Model

Bagozzi, Baumgartener and Pieters [37] analyzed the processes that regulate goal-directed behaviors in the maintenance of healthy weight. According to the authors, the achievement of a goal of weight loss would be explained from the role of anticipatory emotions in positive and negative valence. Depending on the type of emotional advances that prefigures the individual before or during the performance of the lens, there is a different result, which explains the outcome. The authors describe a range of emotions involved in fostering the achievement of a goal in the field of health, i.e. happiness, a sense of satisfaction, guilt, worry, etc. [38].

10 - Bruchon-Schweitzerand and Dantzer Explanatory Model

Even in this model, the nuclear construct is *coping*. However, the coping construct is influenced by perceived stress, received social support, and any existing anxiety state. The first would, in turn, be mediated by certain stressors or life events, and illnesses or unpleasant experiences. Social support is influenced by biological and social factors that characterize the individual, such as age, physical condition, and the family and work situation. The variable of a state of anxiety refers to psychological characteristics; in particular, those that are personality traits and psychological processes inherent to the subject's lifestyle [39].

3. Critical Aspects Related to Bio-Psycho-Social Model

The theoretical references above have provided a significant contribution to health issues since they represent a standard deviation excluding health as the absence of disease, which is why they pertain to the biological aspects, psychological aspects, and social aspects that can influence one's health.

1) Through some theoretical constructs like motivation, intention, and coping effectiveness, we tried to identify the correct explanation of health behavior [40]. We found out that health behavior is related to several different actions, which are collectively called the bio-psycho-social model. However, from an epistemological point of view, the factors that involve biological, psychological, and social aspects belong to different levels. For example, the psychological aspect and the social aspect do not have an empirical reference. They have categorical abstractions, constructs based on hypothetical processes, based strictly on the point of view of the observer. The so-called chemical-biological factors, on the other hand, refer to elements of matter, ontological data, and can be placed on a factual-empirical scale. They are therefore amenable to the logic of cause and effect. Explaining the interactions between factors (in the psychological and social field, they are theoretical constructs), then, means to refer to theoretical hypotheses and to treat them in terms of causality, as if they were objective data. From the epistemological point of view, the interaction between these factors is therefore very critical, as it is built from the mingling of different cognitive levels and used in medical, biological terms [41].

2) The theories described above do not focus on the absence of disease and refer to health through the lens of well-being, used both in political terms (well-being as a human right, 1978 [42]) and in operating terms (as a resource for everyday life, 1986 [43, 44]). The term well-being is composed of the terms "well" and "being." The term "being" is likely to refer to humans in terms of substance, as if they had an "objective body." The adjective "well" is the positive aspect of the word "well-being" - however, it opens up the dichotomy between "well-being" and "ill-being" without defining what "well" and "ill" mean. In conclusion, we witness a further reification (of the term well-being) in an attempt to clarify the meaning of the word health.
3) However, the bio-psycho-social model does not give a clear definition of how to interact with the biological, psychological, and social aspects of health. The definition for health remains uncertain in this model. It is often made to coincide with the idea of healthy behavior, which is related to actions like avoiding smoking and drinking, doing useful examinations, and using condoms. In this way, health remains bound to the behaviors that prevent disease.

Although the bio-psycho-social model has produced notable contributions to health issues and the organizations that deal with them, it is necessary to emphasize that an epistemologically founded definition of health is still absent from it. The implication is that operators are likely to put factual/empirical assumptions within the medical model. In fact, in the medical field, it is possible to empirically detect a normal condition (health) of the body with respect to a pathological one (disease), which authorizes healthcare providers to intervene by removing the cause and obtaining a definite effect (healing). This practice is not acceptable in psychological and social areas, because there is no empirical and objective reference and there is no demonstrable causal relationship between the elements. From this, we can guess how medical practices and culture are still very influential in academic institutions, much more than European definitions allow.

4. TOWARD A CHANGE OF PERSPECTIVE: FROM BIO-PSYCHO-SOCIAL MODEL TO INTERACTIVE-DIALOGICAL MODEL

As was mentioned in the last paragraph, the bio-psycho-social model does not provide enough definition to the object studied and contains epistemologically ambiguous implications; for example, the causal methodology applied to hypothetical and conceptual processes [33, 40, 41, 45, and 46]. It appears in both scientific terms and operational terms. Therefore, it is not an ontological health entity, such as healthcare. It is necessary to clarify references under an epistemic understanding.

5. EPISTEMOLOGICAL AND GNOSEOLOGICAL REFERENCES

Epistemology is a branch of philosophy that concerns the study of the main criteria that distinguish scientific sense from common sense. The term "epistemology" is derived from the Greek "*epistème*" which means "certain knowledge", "foundation", "science" and "*lògos*", i.e. "speech".

There is a similar term, which is "gnoseology ("study of knowledge")", composed from the Greek words "gnosis" and "logos". "Gnosis" always means "knowledge": the Indo-European root "gn-/gen-/gne-/gno" - takes on the meaning of 'notice', 'learning with understanding', 'know something', and then: 'know'. "Episteme" means "certain knowledge" in the sense of knowing a static completed knowledge, as opposed to "gnosis" which mostly refers to "movement". The term "discourse" (λόγος), however, comes from the Greek λέγειν (léghein) meaning "choose", "report", "enumerate"; traditionally, it was considered as the principle that moves things and that makes existence possible[1].

The scientist has to clarify his own studio and define the nature of the knowledge object, in this case health, identifying a given cognitive paradigm, namely a "template", a "project" within which it can be placed for scientific establishment.

[1] C.f. *Enciclopedia Garzanti di Filosofia*, 2004.

The epistemological reflection, which takes as its principle the "logos", is used to identify three levels of realism: monist, hypothetical and conceptual [47].

These three realism levels attempt to answer the questions "What is reality?" and "What is its object?"

The following are the realism levels with all their differences.

1) *Monist realism* considers reality as existing in itself, irrespective of the categories of knowledge of the observer. It claims the priority of "being", of the observed and it is in reference to this epistemological status that science tries to be "neutral" and "objective". The theories are not considered as maps to hypothesize what is ontological, and what is reality, but are considered coincidentally with it. Reality is, therefore, a percept [48]. The sciences which fall within this level of knowledge, such as physics and chemistry, define their object of interest (being) as identified in the ontological level and also measurable (called "ica"). The object's measurability is one of the criteria for demarcating scientific sense from common sense [41]. Common sense says that the sciences that move on the ontological level can be generally defined as exact sciences or "strong" sciences, as they work on the links of cause and effect and are deemed concrete reality.
2) In *hypothetical realism*, reality is not considered a percept, which does not bring in the denotative value of language itself, so as a last resort is not considered at the epistemological level as a 'being' but assumes significant ontological reality of the moment in which it is assumed. The observer is like the one who moves within monistic realism, who considers reality as ontological, but unknowable, except through the formulation of subjective theories; in other words, there are different ways of knowing the same reality. Between knowledge and reality, there is no isomorphism, since the object of investigation is given by the theory of the observer. The concept is developed from the Kantian distinction of noumenon "the thing itself" (unknowable) and phenomenon "as it is known" (known).
3) In *conceptual realism*, reality is not considered on an ontological level, but it is built in the moment in which it is "named". Reality is constructed in the very act of knowing, through the categories of knowledge put into action by one who knows. In summary, the observer creates the reality that he observes. The "how" is known;

> then the process becomes central to this level with respect to the content - i.e. the "what" is known. Therefore, the reality does not exist ontologically and cannot be separated from the theories of those who generate it. The interest is placed on the generation process of the theories, which would be there even without the language [47, 48, 49].

In relation to health, cognitive and epistemological positions are different. If you feel that health exists regardless of the way in which the narrative takes on meaning (or is objective), then you hold a monist position. If we believe we have a theory, then we are faced with hypothetical constructs. If we believe that health is produced by narrative modes and therefore the language inherently defines it, then we are faced with a "reality" concept, i.e. built from the theory of reference, both personal and scientific.

In epistemic terms, therefore, "health" has meaning only within the perspective of hypothetical or conceptual knowledge; otherwise, we would be in front of an objective knowledge, such as "health care" (of the body). "Health" is thus defined by different theories, such as if the individual "speculates" in a different way (hypothetical realism) or he/she "builds" (through a specific narrative) in a different way (conceptual approach). In a conceptual horizon, the health promotion object of investigation is the discursive process [50], through which we build health. The discursive process is a language process with symbolic value [49]. In this sense, what matters most are not the intervening factors in health, but how they find meaning in the narrative of the person. It is therefore necessary to consider narrative links that people use to orient themselves with respect to an action or another person. Consistent with this, health is not the health of the body, but rather a way of life. Health "builds" experience associated with disease, even before it occurs independently of the disease itself. All this creates a gap between health understood in terms of objective health and health understood in the narrative sense. To paraphrase Epictetus, it is not the disease that hurts us, but the idea we have of it.

This highlights the difference between content (some aspects of health) and discursive process (such as the story, as we build it). In this sense, it highlights the need for a paradigm shift, understood through references to Kuhn [51], who argues that scientific development is given by a difference between one way of thinking and another; that it is not realized and instead is understood in cumulative and linear terms. Among the approaches that are most related to the idea that reality is "constructed" is the interactionist approach, within which the construct of identity is key. The construct of identity allows the subject to realize how the "psychological reality" is constructed in interaction with others.

6. The Interactionist Perspective

Deriving some of his assumptions from studies of G.H. Mead [52] and symbolic interactionism studies, a first formalization of the interactionist perspective was defined by Alessandro Salvini [47, 53, 54]. The basic thesis is about the reality "constructed" character, especially starting from the interaction that occurs between two people in a symbolic reference to the context within which they are located.

The interactionist approach considers social processes, be they functional or dysfunctional, as the product of an active construction of meanings by actors in relation to each other and themselves through forms of social negotiation historically contextualized. The main conceptual elements of this perspective can be described as follows:

- People actively generate the experience of suffering from "side effects". People think and act based on the meanings they attach to events, although they are not always aware of what brings out these meanings;
- People build themselves, others and the world experience, even if considered pathological, through representational systems of which language, action and communication are the most important generative elements;
- Representational systems are built by people across social and cultural interaction, and are therefore comprehensible only within the relational contexts that organize and maintain them [55, 56];
- Forms of thought and action problems are not right or wrong, healthy or pathological, but only attempted solutions with adaptive intent and dysfunctional outcomes.

The interactionist perspective attributes a significant role to linguistic and pragmatic, cultural and situational processes through which people construct the forms of their discomfort and their deviant solutions [57, 58, 59].

7. The Construct of Identity

In his essay, *Human Nature and the Social Order,* Cooley (1902) [60] developed the theory of the self as the *Looking-Glass Self*: a theory in which society provides a mirror in which everyone shows his or her true image. In Cooley's system, identity is created in reciprocity of each other. Society can be considered as a mirror in which we see the reactions that others have toward our behavior. This is not a deterministic process; in fact, our identity, according to this theory, does not automatically follow from what others think of us, but the way in which we think we appear to others. Basically, it is what a person sees in the mirror. However, it is never quite the same as we actually appear to others, but it is always the result of a self-reflection and an interpretation of self-recognition.

Referring to the studies of Cooley, G.H. Mead [52], in his book *Mind, Self, and Society* (1934), supports the idea that the self arises from interaction between the individual and society, in the sense that the individual is perceived only by the judgments that other social group members have made about him or her. Identity is something that does not exist at birth but develops as a result of relationships with others and social interaction. The Self of each individual is produced by the interaction between the subject himself and "significant others" that constitute his environment.

For the American sociologist Talcott Parsons [61, 62], a person's identity is in a difficult balance between social and personal components: each person is a child of their own culture and their own society, but also of their specific individualistic experience. This is a central role in the formation of the socialization process that allows the acquisition of guidelines required to deal with the system of expectations related to one or more roles. According to Parsons [63, 64, 65], however, identity is never ultimately achieved, but is a dynamic and open process constructed in interactions; it is constantly changing.

In reference to the conflict between individual and social components, Elias [66, 67] distinguishes between identity - Self (what distinguishes man from other men) - and identity - Us (what he has in common with them). The individual can refer to "Self" only if he/she is able to identify "Us": personal identity has as its preconditions the existence of others and a number of social memberships. If you look at human life in its entirety, it seems difficult to conceive identity in terms of a "me without us." According to the author, the type of relationship between "Self" and "Us" changes in different societies and at different stages of an individual's life.

In the work *The Presentation of the Self in Everyday Life* (1959) by Erving Goffman [68], the metaphor of life as a theater presents a conception of individual identity under which each individual is an actor and the character of a permanent play, set up and rearranged every day, hour by hour, moment by moment. In this sense, identity is structured on the one hand through a continuous development of the Self (the role of the actor), and on the other, through a negotiation of Self in dynamic relationships (the character).

In 1966, Berger and Luckmann [69] argue that the "[s]elf is a reflected entity, reflecting the attitudes of others toward itself." Identity is formed in social processes and social relations in which individuals are involved and are constantly reshaping.

According to the authors, personal identity is formed, preserved, and developed within a web of social relations that has a center. That center is represented by a ring of significant others, those closest and most important to you (spouses, parents, children, colleagues, friends, etc.), and a chorus (distant relatives, colleagues with whom you have less acquaintance, neighbors, acquaintances, etc.).

The relationships between all of these parties contribute daily to confirming, through recognition, to questioning, through criticism, the basic elements of identity.

According to Alessandro Salvini [53], identity can be defined as the result of different psychological processes (intrapersonal and interpersonal skills) resulting in a structure of individual knowledge related to organization of the self. Through personal identity, people have not only cognitive and emotional experiences of themselves but they are also able to: a) develop and integrate in a coherent way the internal and external information that relates to them, such as the somatic and relational (symbolic, expressive and behavioral); b) codify the autobiographical memory form (giving the subjective story a retrospective coherence and future continuity); and c) select and implement behavior repertoires most appropriate to their sexual identity (and gender), developing their socially transmitted skills.

8. The Dialogical Identity Theory

A further development has been defined through the dialogical identity theory from G.P. Turchi. The dialogical identity refers to the discursive process generated by the continuous and constant intersection (dialogical) of three different narrative dimensions: "first person narrator" (*Personalis*), the "expert (*Alter*)" and the "collective matrix (*propter Omnia*)" [41].

a) *Personalis*, or report, which is the set of modes of discourse used by speakers in the definition of their own and others' "health", i.e. the set of discursive productions that fields personal theories about "health".
b) The *Alter*, i.e. discourse modes socially recognized and legitimized as institutionally appointed to define "health" reality, because they enjoy the scientific and institutional recognition, and thus represent an authoritative narrative "voice", particularly pervasive with respect to this definition.
c) *Propter Omnia*, or collective matrix, i.e. the set of discursive modes made available at the historically given socio-cultural context [41].

9. Health as a Dialogic Process and New Paradigmatic Hires

According to this perspective, the way we live and construct "health" is socially and culturally defined, so people construct "greetings" in relation to others. It is for this reason that it is possible to think of "health" in terms of dialogue, differently from conventional approaches to health that often mean "a state." It is generated from the consultation of all the present "narrators" within a specific context. Consistent with the theoretical and epistemological framework adopted, "health" can be defined as a set of modes - discursively understood - that provide for the configuration of reality, in terms of anticipation, the occurrence of diseases, and/or the generation of disease theories [41]

In this sense, it is also possible to describe the difference between health (relative to the body being healthy, or having no diseases) and sanity (the way of promoting the reality "health"), in which the first is considered as a single element of the overall configuration, while the latter is produced by the ways in which a person gives meaning to "health" (narratives).

Starting from the proposed definitions, we can consider that the scope of the relevance of 'health promotion' would cover both configurations of reality that provide for the generation of "disease theories" (according to the diseases for which there are no scientific assumptions of the model doctor, but according to common sense). Both configurations actually contemplate the onset of disease (in this case, health promotion takes care of the discourse processes from which the possibility of acquiring a disease is anticipated, defined as such to an internal medical model).

The relationship is thus to delineate between health psychology and the organic dimension of the disease (and the medical model). It is put in terms of anticipation of possible “future scenarios” that a specific cognitive mode allows you to describe; from the description of a discursive process - therefore, cognitive - that is, it becomes possible to “anticipate” what the same process will allow you to 'build' in terms of the generation of reality; everything should be understood not only as a set of discursive productions related to a “disease theory” but also as pragmatic aspects of the specific construction of reality [41]. In other words, “health” considers "sanity" as a possible situation, which depends on the meaning that is attributed to it, regardless of the severity of the health of the body part affected.

In this sense, the relationship between the onset of disease and the discourse methods used about “health” is not cause and effect, i.e. it is not a deterministic understanding, but it relates to the narrative coherence with which it represents “health.”

According to Prof. Turchi, of the University of Padova, the paradigm that is outlined in this sense is a “narrativistic paradigm” [70] and has the following features:

- First of all, it differs in the work item, which is not content, but the “process of the construction of health”;
- Discourse process is mediated by discursive narrative links, which are rhetorical and argumentative;
- Such narrative links can only be “anticipated,” i.e. seizing the narrative associations people use to carry out an action. Not having an empirical-factual plan, the links cannot be predicted, as is believed in other settings paradigmatic.
- The "work object" is a narrative process with symbolic value; therefore, this process can be changed or maintained. This is very different from "healing": a health care system reference, in which disease and healing exist in an objective way.

Therefore, this switches our understanding of health as a state (or an entity) to a deterministically defined "configuration of reality," with an understood narrative that is procedurally built.

References

[1] Becker, M.H., & Maiman, L.A. (1975). Sociobehavioral determinants of compliance with health and medical care recommendations. *Medical Care,* 13, p. 10-24.

[2] Hochbaum, G.M. (1958). *Public Participation in Medical Screening Programs: A Sociopsychological Study.* US Government Printing Office, Washington, DC.

[3] Rosenstock, I.M. (1974). Historical origins of the health belief model. *Health Education Monographs, 2,* 1–8.

[4] Rogers, R.W., & Prentice-Dunn, S. Protection Motivation Theory. In D. Gochman (ed.), *Handbook of Health Behavior Research. Vol. 1. Determinants of Health Behavior: Personal and Social.* New York: Plenum, 1997.

[5] Maddux, J.E., & Rogers, R.W. (1983). Protection motivation and self efficacy: A revised theory of fear appeals and attitude change. *Journal of Experimental Social Psychology*, 19, 469–479.

[6] Rippetoe, P.A., & Rogers, R.W. (1987). Effects of components of a protection motivation theory on adaptive and maladaptive coping with a health threat. *Journal of Personality and Social Psychology*, 52, 596–604.

[7] Lazarus, R. S. & Folkman. S. (1984). *Stress, appraisal, and coping.* New York: Springer.

[8] Bandura, A. (1977). *Social learning theory.* Englewood Cliffs, NJ: Prentice Hall.

[9] Fishbein, M., & Ajzen, I. (1975). *Belief, attitude, intention, and behavior: An introduction to theory and research.* Reading, MA: Addison-Wesley.

[10] Ajzen, I., & Fishbein, M. (1980). *Understanding attitudes and predicting social behavior.* Englewood Cliffs, NJ: Prentice-Hall.

[11] Sheeran, P. (2002). Intentions-behavior relations: A conceptual and empirical review. In W. Stroebe & M. Hewstone (Eds.). *European Review of Social Psychology,* 12, 1–36.

[12] Conner, M., & Norman, P. (1994). Comparing the health belief model and the theory of planned behaviour in health screening. In D. R. Rutter & L. Quine (Eds.), *Social psychology and health: European perspectives* (pp. 1–24). Aldershot: Avebury.

[13] Conner, M., & Sparks, P. (1996). The theory of planned behaviour and health behaviours. In Conner, M. & Norman, P. (Eds.), *Predicting health behavior.* Buckingham: Open University Press.

[14] Godin, G. (1993). The theories of reasoned action and planned behavior: Overview of findings, emerging research problems and usefulness for exercise promotion. *Journal of Applied Sport Psychology, 5*, p. 141–157.

[15] Murray-Johnson, L., Witte, K., Boulay, M., Figueroa, M.E., Storey, D., & Tweedie, I. (2001) Using health education theories to explain behavior change: a cross-country analysis. *International Quarterly of Community Health Education*, 20, p. 323–345.

[16] Bish, A., Sutton, S. & Golombok, S. (2000) Predicting uptake of a routine cervical smear test: a comparison of the health belief model and the theory of planned behaviour. *Psychology and Health*, 15, 35–50.

[17] Ajzen, I. (1985). From intentions to actions: A theory of planned behavior. In J. Kuhl & J. Beckmann (Eds.), *Action-control: From cognition to behavior* (pp. 11-39). Heidelberg: Springer.

[18] Ajzen, I. (1987). Attitudes, traits, and actions: Dispositional prediction of behavior in personality and social psychology. In Berkowitz, L. (Ed.), *Advances in experimental social psychology*, vol. 20, p. 1-63. New York: Academic Press.

[19] Ajzen, I., & Madden, T. J. (1986). Prediction of goal directed behavior: Attitudes, intentions and perceived behavioral control. *Journal of Experimental Social Psychology*, 22, p. 453–474.

[20] Godin, G., & Kok, G. (1996). The theory of planned behavior: A review of its applications to health-related behaviors. *American Journal of Health Promotion,* 11, p. 87-98.

[21] Schifter, D. B., & Ajzen, I. (1985). Intention, perceived control, and weight loss: An application of the theory of planned behavior. *Journal of Personality and Social Psychology*, 49, p. 843-851.

[22] Terry, D. J., & O'Leary, J. E. (1995). The theory of planned behaviour: the effects of perceived behavioral control and self-efficacy. *British Journal of Social Psychology, 34*, p. 199–220.

[23] Schwarzer, R. (1992). *Self-Efficacy: Thought Control of Action.* Washington, DC: Hemisphere.

[24] Schwarzer, R. & Fuchs, R. (1996). Self-efficacy health behaviors. In M. Conner & P. Norman (Eds.), *Predicting health behavior: Research and practice with social cognition models.* Buckingham: Open University Press.

[25] Bandura, A. (1991). Self-efficacy mechanism in physiological activation and health-promoting behavior. In Madden, J., IV (Ed.), *Neurobiology of learning, emotion and affect* (pp. 229-270). New York: Raven.

[26] Bandura, A. (1992). Self-efficacy mechanism in psychobiologic functioning. In R. Schwarzer (Ed.), *Self-efficacy: Thought control of action* (pp. 355-394). Washington, DC: Hemisphere.

[27] Bandura, A. (1991). Self-efficacy conception of anxiety. In Schwarzer R. & Wicklund R.A. (Eds.), *Anxiety and self-focused attention* (pp. 89-110). New York: Harwood.

[28] Prochaska, J.O., & DiClemente, C.C. (1983). Stages and processes of self-change of smoking: toward an integrative model of change. *Journal of Consulting and Clinical Psychology*, 51 (3), p. 390-5.

[29] Prochaska, J.O., & DiClemente, C.C. (1986). Toward a comprehensive model of change. In Miller, W.R., & Heather, N., *Treating addictive behaviors: processes of change*. New York: Plenum Press.

[30] Prochaska, J.O., & DiClemente, C.C. (1992). Stages of change in the modification of problem behaviors. *Progress in Behavior Modification*, 28, p. 183-218.

[31] Prochaska, J.O., DiClemente, C.C., & Norcross, J.C. (1992). In search of how people change. Applications to addictive behaviors. *American Psychologist*, Sep, 47 (9), p. 1102-14.

[32] Bridle, C., Riemsma, R.P., Pattenden, J., Sowden, A.J., Mather, L., Watt, I.S. & Walker, A. (2005). Systematic rewiew of the effectiveness of health behavior interventions based on the transtheoretical model. *Psychology & Health*, 20, p. 283-301.

[33] Tartarotti, L. (2010). *Psicologia della salute: un'introduzione*. Milano: Franco Angeli.

[34] Prochaska, J.O., & Velicer, W.F. (1997). The transtheoretical model of health behavior change. *American Journal of Health Promotion*, Sep-Oct, 12 (1), p. 38-48.

[35] Rutter, D.R., Quine, L., & Chesham, D.J. (1995). Predicting safe riding behaviour and accidents: demography, beliefs, and behavior in motorcycling safety. *Psychology & Health*, 10, p. 369-386.

[36] Conner, M., & Norman, P. (1996). *Predicting health behaviour*. Buckingham: Open University Press.

[37] Bagozzi, R. P., Baumgartner, H., & Pieters, R. (1998). Goal-directed emotions. *Cognition and Emotion*, 12, 1–26.

[38] Soscia, I. (2007). Gratitude, Delight, or Guilt: The Role of Consumers Emotions in Predicting Postconsumption Behaviors. *Psychology and Marketing,* 24(10), p. 871–894.
[39] Bruchon-Schweitzer, M., Dantzer, R. (1994). *Introduction à la Psychologie de la Santé*. Paris: PUF.
[40] Stroebe, W. (2000). *Social psychology and health.* Philadelphia: Open University Press.
[41] Turchi, G.P., & Della Torre, C., (2007). *Psicologia della salute - dal modello bio-psico-sociale al modello dialogico: generare e gestire processi trasformativi nell'ambito della "salute"*. Roma: Armando.
[42] World Health Organization. (1978). *Declaration of Alma-Ata: International conference on primary health care, Alma-Ata, USSR, 6–12 September 1978.* Retrieved February 14, 2006, from http://www.who.int/hpr/NPH/docs/ declaration_almaata.pdf
[43] World Health Organization. (1986). *The Ottawa charter. Geneva:* World Health Organization.
[44] Bognar, G. (2008). Well-being and health. *Health Care Analysis*, 16, p. 97-113.
[45] Bertini, M. (2012). *Psicologia della Salute*. Roma: Raffaello Cortina.
[46] Antonovsky, A. (1996). The salutogenic model as a theory to guide health promotion. *Health Promotion International,* 11 (1), p. 11–18.
[47] Salvini A. (1998). *Argomenti di Psicologia Clinica*. Padova: Upsel-Domeneghini.
[48] Salvini A. (1992). Pluralismo teorico e pragmatismo conoscitivo: assunti metateorici in psicologia della personalità. In Fiora, E., Pedrabissi, L., Salvini, A., *Pluralismo teorico e pragmatismo conoscitivo in psicologia della personalità*. Milano: Giuffré.
[49] Wittgenstein, L. (1953). *Philosophical Investigations*. Oxford: Blackwell.
[50] Harrè R., & Gillett G. (1994). *The discursive mind.* Thousand Oaks: Sage.
[51] Kuhn, T. (1969). *La struttura delle rivoluzioni scientifiche*. Torino: Einaudi.
[52] Mead, G.H. (1934). *Mind, self and society*. Chicago: University of Chicago Press.
[53] Salvini, A., Ravasio, A., & Da Ros, T. (2008). *Psicologia clinica giuridica*. Firenze: Giunti.
[54] Salvini, A., & Dondoni, M. (2011). *Psicologica clinica dell'interazione*. Firenze: Giunti.

[55] Faccio, E., Fusa, V., Iudici, A. (2013). New Ideas for health promotion programs contrasting eating disorders at schools. *European Journal of Social Behaviour*, vol. V (2), p. 1024-1031.

[56] Faccio, E., Fusa, V., Iudici, A. (2013). When Informing About Eating Disorders Exacerbates the Problem Instead of Preventing it: Which Programs Work and Which Ones do not? *The European Journal of Counselling Psychology*, vol. 2 (2), p. 111-119.

[57] Faccio, E. (2012). *The Corporeal Identity: When the Self-Image Hurts*. New York: Springer.

[58] Salvini, A., Iudici, A., & Mazzini C. (2011). La psicoterapia interazionista: presupposti e prassi clinica. In *Psicologia Clinica dell'Interazione e Psicoterapia*, (a cura di Dondoni M., Salvini A.), Ed. Firenze: Giunti, p. 300-313.

[59] *Dizionario di Psicologia e Psicoterapia*, (cura di), Nardone G., Salvini A. (2012) Ed. Garzanti.

[60] Cooley, C. H. (1964). *Human nature and the social order*. New York: Schocken Books. (Original work published 1902).

[61] Parsons, T. (1937). *The Structure of Social Action: a study in social theory with special reference to a group of recent European writers*. New York: McGraw-Hill.

[62] Parsons, T. (1939). *Action, Situation and Normative Pattern: An Essay in the Theory of Social Action*. Wien: LIT.

[63] Parsons, T. (1951). *The Social System*. Routledge and Kegan Paul Ltd.

[64] Parsons, T. (1954). *Essays in Sociological Theory*. New York: Free Press.

[65] Parsons, T. (1960). *Structure and Process in Modern Societies*. New York: John Wiley.

[66] Elias, N. (1939). *Über den Prozeß der Zivilisation. Soziogenetische und psychogenetische Untersuchungen. Erster Band. Wandlungen des Verhaltens in den weltlichen Oberschichten des Abendlandes* and *Zweiter Band. Wandlungen der Gesellschaft. Entwurf einer Theorie der Zivilisation*. Basel: Verlag Haus zum Falken. (Published in English as *The Civilizing Process, Vol. I. The History of Manners*, Oxford: Blackwell, 1969, and *The Civilizing Process, Vol. II. State Formation and Civilization*, Oxford: Blackwell, 1982).

[67] Elias, N., & Scotson, J. (1965). *The Established and the Outsiders. A Sociological Enquiry into Community Problems*. London: Frank Cass & Co.

[68] Goffman, E. (1959). *The Presentation of Self in Everyday Life*. London: Penguin.

[69] Berger P.L. & Luckmann T. (1966). *The Social Construction of Reality: A Treatise its the Sociology of Knowledge*. Garden City, New York: Anchor Books, 1966, pp. 51-61. Trad. it. Berger, P., Luckman, T. (1969). *La realtà come costruzione sociale*. Bologna: il Mulino.

[70] Turchi, G. P., Durante, R., & Perno, A. (2002). Verso un paradigma narrativistico. In G. P. Turchi (A cura di), "*Tossicodipendenza". Generare il cambiamento tra mutamento di paradigma ed effetti pragmatici* (p. 103-117). Padova: Upsel.

Chapter 3

HEALTH PROMOTION IN SCHOOL: CONCEPTUAL ASSUMPTIONS

1. INTRODUCTION

Among the places for health promotion, school occupies a special place. School is a place where students are taught how to be sensible to this topic. Everywhere in the world, different themes are treated in schools, such as sexual education, bullying, preventions against drug abuse, racism etc. [1, 2].

There are many reasons for intervening in schools; first, there is the need to intercept the youth segment of the population before the convictions of young people themselves become very structured [4]. In school, the first beliefs and opinions grow that will turn into real theories. By hosting the student for a number of hours weekly, and for a very long period, the school may have a significant role in monitoring what "existential" model the student is constructing; whether it be a mindset of health or one of tending disease. Often, young people's beliefs are those of the adults who attend more, who are often members of their own family. This offers the possibility to intercept what adults think about health and especially how they contribute to constructing it.

2. THE SCHOOL AS STRATEGY

Intervention in school thus becomes a strategic action to be taken toward adults, as well as a hub of the community as a whole.

In addition, the involvement of the school is important because:

a) There is acknowledgement of some topics that might not be talked about at home, like sexually transmitted diseases.
b) The setting facilitates the acquisition of civil rules, concepts, or concerns that might otherwise be acquired in informal environments such as knowledge of certain rules or social offenses for foreign students.
c) It allows for establishing interpersonal relationships independently of the family, teachers, principals and school staff.
d) It can support the students by addressing issues that do not relate to the school but can nevertheless affect performance.
e) The school can facilitate contact with other institutions in order to share and exchange methodologies.
f) It provides the opportunity to intervene with people surrounding the young people e.g. parents, teachers etc.
g) The school helps to interpret the promotion of health, regarding its role and the students' responsibility for it [5].

3. Difficulties of Working in the School

Despite the merits of those reasons, working in schools on topics that are not strictly educational is not always easy. First, this is because institutions that deal with young people have different goals; except in some states, the school has only educational goals, while institutions that deal with health-related targets are oriented toward healthy behavior.

There are also a number of other difficulties, including that of identifying a shared plan between outside professionals and teachers. It is often difficult to find time and space to create a permanent strategy, both in terms of design [6, 7] and valuation [8, 9]. In many cases, there is no willingness on the part of teachers to deal with issues that are not purely academic. This often means the distorted beliefs that teachers and leaders sometimes have toward health are not intercepted [10]. In some cases, there are no agreements between the Ministry of Health and the Ministry of Education, and this leads to the activation of local initiatives, which are sporadic and based on the personal inclination of the individual manager. Initiatives for students usually take place without either involving students themselves, or they are performed in the same environments as daily lessons, thus producing interventions that resemble informative lessons [11, 12]. From this, we create the conditions for students to live the school experience in terms of income.

Despite the World Health Organization, WHO [13, 14] having demonstrated the key role that some institutions can have, such as ministries of health and education at the national level, and non-governmental organizations at the local level, another critical aspect concerns the ineffectiveness of the interaction between the institutions that deal with health [15, 16]. In particular, there seems to be a lack of knowledge of school organizations [17, 18, 19, 20].

Willke [21] introduced the term "contextual approach" in reference to the need to consider the capacity for self-organization of schools and support their development relative to their own objectives. In this sense, schools are to be considered complex organizational systems [16], different from each other according to their own history and their own identity [22, 23].

4. Health Promotion Interventions in the School

With regard to health promotion interventions implemented in the school, the international literature highlights much evidence, both in relation to specific issues and to methodological issues [24, 25, 26, 27]. For the first case, health promotion is applied in the context of nutrition and healthy eating [28, 29, 30, 31, 32], as part of sexuality [33, 34, 35], in the context of sanitation [34], within the context of substance abuse [37, 38, 39], physical activity [40, 41, 42] and dementia [43]. Even just the areas mentioned can be understood in terms of the promotion intervention being still inextricably linked to the treatment of specific themes or content.

At the same time the health promotion interventions attempt to approach the school in global terms [44, 45, 46, 47, 48], although there is not a precise definition of what it can mean for the global economy. However, some of the directions that appear most shareable are:

- The intervention is oriented to the school context and not to the individual
- The intervention must be consistent with school policies
- The intervention must actively involve school staff, students, teachers and other roles, both in terms of design and for the final evaluation
- The intervention must encourage the development of skills in students and teachers and develop the participation of the whole school community

- The intervention will assist the school in achieving its goals [1].

Despite the intentions described above and the results achieved, it is necessary to remember that health promotion activities are not widespread today in all countries [49, 50, 51]. Moreover, in many countries, interventions are aimed at reducing the factors related to the disease (or risk), directly and indirectly. In other countries, other approaches to health promotion are used. However, we often relate health topics to dysfunctions of the body (then still associated with the disease). Most of the experiences of health promotion have reified the concept of health.

In many contexts, the following definition is used:

> "Health promotion in the school context can be defined as any activity undertaken to improve and/or protect the health of all stakeholders in the school community, and in this sense implies (...) policies for a healthy school, school environments as places of physical and social, educational curricula for health, links and joint activities with other services directed to citizens and health services" [1].

The definition mentioned above does not specify what is meant by health, and the term health is reified, as if health was an objective fact. Implicitly, it refers to the dysfunctions of the body and, as we have already seen, we consider the factors that may explain the behaviors that produce them. We are now going to review some topics in which a change of perspective is particularly urgent: smoking, delinquency, bullying, and interculturality.

REFERENCES

[1] St Leger, L., Blanchard, C., Perry, M., & Young, I. (2010). *Promoting Health in Schools: from Evidence to Action.* France: International Union for Health Promotion and Education.

[2] McQueen, D.V. & Jones, C.M. (2007). *Global Perspectives on Health Promotion Effectiveness.* New York: Springer Science & Business Media.

[3] Lister-Sharp, D., Chapman, S., Stewart-Brown, S., & Sowden, A. (1999). Health promoting schools and health promotion in schools: Two systematic reviews. *Health Technology Assessment*, 3, p. 1-207.

[4] De Santi, A., Guerra, R., & Morosini, P. (2008). *La promozione della salute nelle scuole: obiettivi di insegnamento e competenze comuni.* Roma: Superiore di Sanità (Rapporti ISTISAN 08/1).

[5] Pearson, M., Chilton, R. Woods, H.B., Wyatt, K., Ford, T., Abraham, C., & Anderson, R. (2012). Implementing health promotion in schools: protocol for a realist systematic review of research and experience in the United Kingdom (UK). *Systematic Reviews*, 1 (1), p. 48.

[6] Bonell, C., Harden, A., Wells, H., Jamal, F., Fletcher, A., Petticrew, M., & Moore, L. (2011). Protocol for a systematic review of the effects of schools and school-environment interventions on health: evidence mapping and syntheses. *BMC public health*, 11 (1), p. 453.

[7] Bonell, C., Fletcher, A., Morton, M., Lorenc, T., & Moore, L. (2012). Realist randomised controlled trials: A new approach to evaluating complex public health interventions. *Social Science & Medicine,* 75, p. 2299-2306.

[8] Pawson, R., Owen, L., & Wong, G. (2010). The Today Programme's Contribution to Evidence based Policy. *Evaluation*, 16, p. 211-214.

[9] Pawson, R. & Tilley, N. (1997). *Realistic Evaluation.* London: Sage Publications. www.iuhpe.org, accessed 20 June, 2009.

[10] St. Leger, L. (2005). Protocols and guidelines for health promoting schools. *Promotion & Education,* 12 (3-4), p. 145–147.

[11] International Union for Health Promotion (2007) *Strategic directions 2007–2013* [Internet]. IUHPE Paris, France. 2007. Available from: www.iuhpe.org, accessed 20 June, 2009.

[12] Barnekow Rasmussen, V., Burgher, M.S. & Rivett, D. (1999). *The European Network of Health Promoting Schools – the alliance of education and health.* 16-18, Conference Resolution, Thessaloniki 1-5 May, 1997. WHO Regional Office for Europe/ European Commission / Council of Europe.

[13] World Health Organization (2005). *Strategy for child and adolescent health and development*, draft to be presented to the Regional Committee September 2005.

[14] World Health Organization (2007). *Schools for Health, Education and Development: A Call for Action*. Geneva: World Health Organization.

[15] Denman, S., Moon, A., Parsons, C. & Stears, D. (2002) *The Health Promoting School- Policy Research and Practice.* London: Routledge.

[16] Keshavarz, N., Nutbeam, D., Rowling, L., Khavarpour, F. (2010). Schools as social complex adaptive systems: a new way to understand

the challenges of introducing the health promoting schools concept. *Social Science & Medicine*, 70, p. 1467-74.

[17] MacDonald, M. A., & Green, L. W. (2001). Reconciling concept and context: The dilemma of implementation in school-based health promotion. *Health Education & Behavior,* 28 (6), p. 749-768.

[18] Land, D. (2002). Local school boards under review: their role and effectiveness in relation to students' academic achievement. *Review of Educational Research*, vol. 72 (2), p. 229-78.

[19] Alvesson, M. & Sveningsson, S. (2003a). Good visions, bad micro-management and ugly ambiguity: Contradictions of (non-) leadership in a knowledge-intensive organization. *Organization Studies, 24*(6), 961-988. DOI: 10.1177/0170840603024006007.

[20] Shiell, A., Hawe, P., & Gold, L. (2008). Complex interventions or complex systems? Implications for health economic evaluation. *British Medical Journal*, 336, p. 1281–1283

[21] Willke, H. (2007). *Smart Governance: Governing the Global Knowledge Society. Frankfurt am Main.* New York: Campus-Verlag.

[22] Cilliers, P. (1998). *Complexity and Postmodernism: Understanding Complex Systems.* London: Routledge.

[23] Lange S., & Schimank, U. (2004). A political sociology for complex societies: Niklas Luhmann. In: Nash, K., & Scott, A. *The Blackwell Companion to Political Sociology.* Oxford, UK & Australia: Blackwell Publishing, Carlton.

[24] Gugglberger, L. (2011). Support for health promoting schools: a typology of supporting strategies in Austrian provinces. *Health Promot. Int.*, 26 (4), p. 447-456.

[25] Jensen, B.B. & Simovska, V. (eds) (2002). *Models of Health Promoting Schools in Europe.* WHO Regional Office for Europe, Copenhagen.

[26] Stewart-Brown, S. (2006). *What is the evidence on school health promotion in improving school health or preventing disease and specifically what is the effectiveness of the health promoting schools approach?* Copenhagen: World Health Organization.

[27] Gugglberger, L., & Dur, W. (2011). Capacity building in and for health promoting schools: results from a qualitative study. *Health Policy*, 101 (1), p. 37–43.

[28] Lobstein, T., & Swinburn, B. (2007). Health Promotion to Prevent Obesity: Evidence and Policy Needs. In McQueen, D., & Jones, C. *Global perspective on Health.* New York: Springer Science & Business Media.

[29] Faccio, E., Fusa, V., & Iudici, A. (2013). New Ideas for health promotion programs contrasting eating disorders at schools. *European Journal Of Social Behaviour*, vol. V, (2), p. 1024-1031.

[30] Faccio, E., Fusa, V., & Iudici, A. (2013). When Informing About Eating Disorders Exacerbates the Problem Instead of Preventing it: Which Programs Work and Which Ones do not? *The European Journal of Counselling Psychology*, vol. 2 (2), p. 111-119.

[31] Perry, C.L., Luepker, R.V., Murray, D.M., Kurth, C., Mullis, R., Crockett, S., & Jacobs, D.R. Jr. (1988). Parent involvement with children's health promotion: the Minnesota Home Team. *American Journal of Public Health,* 78, 9, p. 1156-1160.

[32] Campbell, C., Waters, E., O'Meara, S. & Summerbell, C. (2001). Interventions for preventing obesity in childhood. A systematic review. *Obesity Reviews: An official journal of the International Association for the Study of Obesity*, Aug, 2 (3), p. 149-57.

[33] Kirby, D. (2002). The impact of schools and school programs upon adolescent sexual behavior. *Journal of Sex Research*, 39 (1), p. 27-33.

[34] Young Song E., Pruitt, B., McNamara, J. & Colwell, B. (2000). A meta-analysis Examining Effects of School Sexuality Education Programs on Adolescents' Sexual Knowledge, 1960–1997. *Journal of School Health*, 70 (10), p. 412-416.

[35] Silva, M. (2002). The effectiveness of school-based sex education programs in the promotion of abstinent behaviour: a meta-analysis. *Health Education Research*, 17, (4), p. 471-481.

[36] Brian, A. & Haggard, S. (2003). *Hygiene Promotion: Evidence and Practice.* London: School of Hygiene and Tropical Medicine.

[37] McBride, N. (2003). A systematic review of school drug education. *Health Education Research*, 18 (6), p. 729-742.

[38] Stead, M., & Angus, K. (2004). Literature review into the effectiveness of school drug education. *Scottish Executive, August.*

[39] Thomas, R., (2002). School-based programmes for preventing smoking. *The Cochrane Database of Systematic Reviews*, 4, Art. No. CD001293, p. 149-147.

[40] Timperio, A., Salmon, J., & Ball, K. (2004). Evidence-based strategies to promote physical activity among children, adolescents and young adults: review and update. *Journal of Science and Medicine in Sport,* 7 (1), p. 20-29.

[41] Sibley, B.A., & Etnier, J.L. (2003). The relationship between physical activity and cognition in children: A meta-analysis. *Pediatric Exercise Science*, 15, p. 243-256.

[42] van Beurden, E., Barnett, L.M., Zask, A., Dietrich, U.C., Brooks, L.O., & Beard, J. (2003). Can we skill and activate children through primary school physical education lessons? "move it groove it"- a collaborative health promotion intervention. *Preventive Medicine*, 36 (4), p. 493-501.

[43] Belloni E., Faccio E., Costa N., & Iudici A. (2014) Health professionals working with persons with Dementia. Reflections for new training courses. *Procedia- Social Behavioral Sciences*, vol. 116, p. 4700-4705.

[44] ENHPS (1997). *Conference Resolution. First Conference of the European Network of Health Promoting Schools.* WHO Regional office for Europe, Copenhagen.

[45] Jensen, B. & Simovska, V. (2002). *Models of Health Promoting Schools in Europe. ENHPS Technical Secretariat, Copenhagen*, WHO Regional Office for Europe.

[46] IUHPE (2008). *Achieving Health Promoting Schools: Guidelines for Promoting Health in Schools,* 2nd ed., International Union for Health Promotion and Education, Geneva.

[47] IUHPE (2009). *Promoting Health in Schools: From Evidence to Action.* International Union for Health Promotion and Education, Geneva.

[48] St Leger, L., Kolbe, L., Lee, A., McCall, D., & Young, I. (2007). School health promotion: Achievements, challenges and priorities. Chapter in D. McQueen, & Jones C. (2007). *Global perspectives in health promotion effectiveness*. New York: Springer Science & Business Media.

[49] Deschesnes, M., Martin, C., & Hill, A.J. (2003). Comprehensive approaches to school promotion: how to achieve broader implementation? *Health Promotion International*, 18 (4), p. 387-396.

[50] Glasgow R.E., Lichtenstein E., & Marcus A.C. (2003). Why don't we see more translation of health promotion research to practice? Rethinking the efficacy-to-effectiveness transition. *American Journal of Public Health,* 93, p. 1261-1267.

[51] Clift S., Jensen B. B. Colquhoun D. (2005). Complexity and the health promoting school. In: Clift, S., Jensen, B.B. *The Health Promoting School: International Advances in Theory, Evaluation and Practice.* Copenhagen: Danish University of Education Press, p. 41-53.

PART TWO

Chapter 4

TOBACCO AND SCHOOLS: HISTORICAL REFERENCES, CONCEPTS AND METHODS OF INTERVENTION

1. INTRODUCTION

In this chapter we will discuss the measures taken against the use of tobacco in school. Such a theme is of great significance, first and foremost because of the involvement of remarkable sanitarian issues, and secondly since the act of smoking tends to be a "normal" custom among many teenagers, and because the consumption of cigarettes, although also performed by adults, most frequently causes implicit contrasts, conflicts and disagreements between young people and adults [1].

In most cases, the act of smoking is done as part of group and family dynamics that are often even more complex than they seem, especially when a young person starts to smoke. Among the family group, the smoking parents provide a model in which the younger members can relate, even if the parents might verbally disagree with this model. Non-smoking parents can find themselves in the opposite situation, by attempting to persuade their children not to smoke; hence, struggles over control and moral implications take place and often resolve themselves in a radicalization of the different points of view. Outside the family setting, it is well known that the act of smoking is often related to factors such as peers, bonds of friendship and group dynamics. It is in such situations that the consumption of tobacco is established.

As has been noticed, the act of smoking itself is not only a practical action but it has also a valuable social and existential meaning. As a matter of fact, it often implies some other and more complex processes, such as self-representation, the feeling of belonging to a group and the creation of one's own personal identity. In this case, it quickly becomes evident as well that the discussion about this theme at school has wide appeals and repercussions that go beyond the mere learning process.

Intervening with students at school means an attempt to shape the future citizens and, once again, the institution of the school represents the background in which social requirements are conducted, such as developing a greater sense of health care in younger people. Such an assignment, however, is not adequately supported in terms of financial investments and in most cases the school is unable to properly satisfy the requests. Therefore, it is necessary to provide schools (all those that deal with health care) with all the resources and competences needed to face all the questions that society asks them to address.

As regards the consumption of tobacco, the research has moreover highlighted the lack of effectiveness of the interventions implemented thus far; mostly, these have been centered on interventions regarding "behavior". Complications involve several aspects: first, training for teachers is not widespread. Moreover, in many cases the "addiction" cannot be considered as "evident", as adolescence is characterized by a clearly unstable behavior. Furthermore, the influence of multinational tobacco companies in promoting the spread of smoking behavior among people makes it harder for school institutions to achieve their goal.

2. Reference Standards

Given that regulatory references promoted by WHO were presented in the previous chapters, hereinafter what was made available by the European Union will be presented. What we are interested in is not a focus on the European context, but instead it is the extraction of technical and conceptual references utilized by regulations. The first legislation of the European Union in the matter of Tobacco Addiction was 89/622/CEE [2], which referred to the priority requirement of decreasing cancers, and stated that "it is very important to ensure the health protection of individuals, to place on the packaging material of every product of tobacco an advisory stressing the risks for the health". It was also necessary to specify the "import of tar and nicotine". It also prohibited the sale of "certain types of tobacco for oral use in every country except for the Kingdom of Sweden, which obtained a waiver".

Noticeably, the approach taken was one of guidance, implicitly expressing the idea that informing consumers (or potential ones) could modify their behavior.

The legislation 90/239/CEE [3], which followed, focuses the attention on the quantity of nicotine and tar in cigarettes, establishing thresholds for these substances according to the ISO/FTC standards. This is a kind of toxicological intervention and contains some critical implications, either because this is merely a medical intervention (distancing itself from the priorities defined by the new definitions of health), or because, even on medical grounds, the biological necessity of smokers who need to maintain a constant level of nicotine in their blood is not taken into account. In fact, several researchers [4] assert that while it seems to be a positive act, instead, it can lead to a progressive increase of the consumption of cigarettes by consumers in order to keep the constant level of nicotine they are used to. All of this could entail the risk of promoting or even legitimizing the usage of "low tar cigarettes", improperly considering them to be less dangerous than the others.

The legislation 92/41/CEE [5], on the basis of the preceding 89/622/CEE [2], reviews some of its articles banning the consumption of some kinds of tobacco for oral use, with the exception of smoking tobaccos and chewing tobaccos which are entirely or partially constituted of tobacco, for which the danger to the health must be highlighted on the packaging with specific advice. Even if such regulation attempts to reduce some social incoherence in prohibiting some products and selling others that are similar, in this case the intention of the intervention is prohibitionist as well.

The most effective legislation was paradoxically the 95/59/CE [6] whose purpose was merely to level the taxation on manufactured tobacco in the European territory; this legislation was reviewed with the legislation 1999/81/CE [7], which led to the increase in the prices of cigarette packs. The basis of it is the research data demonstrating the correlation between the rise in the cost of tobacco and the reduction of its usage [8]. This is especially useful in the case of an adolescent smoker, who, having limited financial resources, would give up smoking. Despite all of this, the price of cigarette packs is different among European countries and this situation seems to foster the trade of illegally imported tobaccos. In 2005 in Italy, the government increased the excise tax on fine-cut tobacco since, due to the rise in prices, consumers became drawn to the "roll your own" tobaccos [9]. The legislation 2001/37/CE [10] is a summary and a connection point of all the preceding legislation. It concerns legislative measures, either regulatory or administrative, of the Member States concerning the manufacturing, launch and trade of tobacco products. In this legislation, it is evident that producers do not provide information about the additives utilized and that this issue prevents the establishment of the overall toxicity level of the product. Information provided on cigarette packages often concerns the percentage of nicotine and tar and for this reason, especially in the past, labels such as "light" or "mild" appeared. Such information is of little use to the consumer, who could be led to think that a "light" cigarette pack would be less dangerous for the health than a pack on which this label doesn't appear. This led people to the use of "light" cigarettes as an alternative to quitting smoking. For all these reasons it was thought that the percentages of substances and labels as "light" and "mild" should be removed from the packs in favor of more useful and accurate information such as the concentration of carcinogenic and other toxins instead of nicotine, and that clear messages should be put on the cover of the pack or in a package leaflet [4]. Returning to legislation, this stressed the importance of having a list of permitted ingredients and in the meantime, the need of Member States to obtain toxicological data on elements implied in the production, in order to have a better idea of the toxicity of such products [10].

3. The Consumption of Tobacco: Research Contributions and Clinical Implications

At the moment the World Health Organization (WHO) estimates that habitual consumers of tobacco number around 1 billion people [11, 12, 13, 14, 15], of which 12% are male adolescents and 7% are female adolescents [16, 17]. It has been observed that tobacco has a strong correlation with neoplasm, cardiovascular and respiratory diseases, and that the deaths caused by smoking habits amount to 6 million per year; it is predicted that by 2030 they will cost about 10 million euros per year [18, 19]. More than 80% of smokers live in a country with low mean per capita [20]; intoxication from tobacco is therefore considered one of the main causes of preventable disease. The effects of tobacco consumption concern either the medical/healthcare area [21, 22] or the psychological area [23, 24]. Many researchers have found that there is a greater correlation between the behavior of people affected by psychological weaknesses and the behavior of non-smoking people, whether it is considered either as the cause or the effect [25, 26]. Other researchers found that nicotine addiction affects psychiatric patients more than the rest of the population, especially patients with schizophrenic syndrome [27]. Some others noticed the existence of a correlation between depressive syndrome, anxiety [26], the inability to control oneself [28] and many other problems concerning pregnancy [29, 30].

For this reason as well, as described in the preceding chapters, the World Health Organization, whose purpose is "*to promote the realization of the highest attainable standard of human health*" [31], aims to fight against the smoking habit; this is the same aim as that of the European Union, one of whose first assignments is "*to protect and to enhance human health*" [32].

4. Fighting Tobacco Addiction at School

After seeing how the consumption of tobacco is hindered by legislation and after having pointed out the general data on the phenomenon, now we are going to see how all of this influences the lives of adolescents and the school environment. The scientific community may disagree, but the idea that smoking initiation begins first in adolescence, especially before the age of 15, is widely shared [33, 34, 35].

Accordingly, the school environment becomes the major context in which one can intervene with that age group, especially for the following reasons: one can easily access a large number of students; it enables one to nip in the bud an activity which can easily became an enduring habit; and one can intercept and involve students' families to establish a collaboration between teachers and local services [36, 37]. Indeed, it is during this stage of life that the majority of interventions against tobacco addiction are conducted.

Historically, the first interventions were in the nineteen-seventies and aimed to inform students about the consequences of cigarette consumption, mostly causing health damage. These interventions were often full of moral judgments and their goal was to threaten smokers and potential smokers. The main message conveyed through the media was: if you know it, you will avoid it. The premise was to hinder the act of smoking through good common sense or "logic", for instance: 'if you know that it hurts, you are not going to do that again'. It quickly became evident that knowing the effects of smoking didn't mean necessarily one would change one's behavior, as every smoker knows well. Indeed, such an approach is nowadays considered ineffective. Later, the behavior of smokers was classified in different psychological categories, such as self-esteem, intention, motivation and emotions [38]. However, this method could not lead to the long-awaited change either [39].

Several research studies have attempted to verify the effectiveness of school projects through meta-analysis to find out remarkable factors.

The results are not unique, even if the major tendency is to consider them as ineffective [40, 41, 42, 43, 44]. There are many reasons for this, but mostly a combination of different approaches and implicit ideas on the interventions have been employed [45, 46, 47]. In many cases, the projects are not valuable, because their purposes are neither valid nor shared [48]. Many interventions aim to modify the "behavior" of the individuals considered at risk [49, 50, 51, 52, 53, 54]. Interventions based on the passage of information are deemed ineffective, whereas social interventions, based on influencing peers, are considered more effective [35, 55, 56].

Based on these data, new interpretations of the phenomenon, especially about a context that requires appropriate analysis, tools and methods to address young people, are needed.

Firstly, let us have a look at the crucial differences between the various intervention approaches to tobacco addiction.

5. Approaches to Tobacco Addiction

In the aforementioned legislation, some of the methods of the approaches to tobacco addiction can be seen: for instance, the interventions aimed at modifying the behavior vs. interventions, aimed at developing particular skills.

5.1. Interventions Aimed at Modifying the Behavior

The purpose of this approach is merely to change the behavior of individuals; it is based on an attempt at modifying the behavior of others. All the activities and projects are oriented to the modification of what is considered to be negative, improper and wrong, be it an attempt to reduce the consumption of cigarettes, avoid the consumption of alcohol, perform control screening, use a condom, etc. It is very important to point out that the act is considered negative by an external observer, not by the person performing the act. That specific action is considered, by definition, egodystonic, in that the way of thinking of the individual who is feeling it is irrelevant. By the latter reference as well, it is possible to recognize the influence of the medical model that tends to objectify the other.

5.1.1. Harm Reduction

Harm reduction is a type of intervention especially widespread in the '80s; its goal is to reduce the aftereffects of the use of a substance considered harmful. This intervention is based on practical activities, which consist in making available for consumers materials (such as information brochures, syringes, and tampons) and tools to promote a risk-mitigation. Such activities very often are implemented in places where substances are normally consumed; for instance, around clubs, campsites and equipped buses. Even if there are several dynamics for the harm reduction to be conducted, there can be two main assumptions on which the strategy is grounded. Firstly, hindering the consumption is not the priority; what matters is instead reducing its consequences. Secondly, every demand for transformation or discouragement of consumption is left. "Consumption rooms" or "shooting rooms" constitute an example of harm reduction because it is possible to use the substances under medical supervision. Every method which allows reducing the aftereffects of substances can fit within the logic of harm reduction. Tools such as cigarette holders, cigarette filters, delivery system nicotine or substances such as chewing tobacco or Swedish snus[1] are often used following the harm reduction logic [57].

5.1.2. Prohibition

In this context, the term prohibition indicates the disqualification of the consumption or sale of certain substances, in order to preserve the health of citizens. Each approach aims to avoid, prevent, reject and ban a specific unhealthy or risk behavior. There can be various forms of prohibition: some forbid the sale and the trade of the substance; others also forbid the consumption of the substance, leading to administrative, civil or criminal consequences, so-called "zero tolerance". Nowadays in different parts of the world there are regulations whose aim is to prohibit tobacco, alcohol, cannabis, cocaine, etc.

5.1.3 Information Approach (Information Living Model)

One of the most common methods within the sanitarian and school system is the transmission of contents. The purpose is to inform the population about

[1] Swedish word for a sort of tobacco coming from different parts of the world, air-dried. It can be powdered or in sachets and it is used by placing it between the upper lip and the gingiva. It can be kept in the mouth for a few minutes or several hours by means of steam humidification.

risks. In many schools and educational settings, activities which aim to highlight the consequences of consumption are preferred. Referring to tobacco addiction, cardiovascular and pulmonary diseases, as well as a number of risks for the body and mind are mentioned, all by means of ex-cathedra lessons, conferences, booklets, brochures, face-to-face lectures, etc. All these procedures need to be objective, neutral, and impartial and need to avoid prejudice.

The implicit requirements of such a model concern: a) the idea of an objective communication, free of the influence of the informer, and b) the certainty that greater information could lead to a modification of attitude and behavior toward the consumption. The effectiveness of the first requirement is denied by studies which see communication as a circular process [58] and by studies which support the idea that it is impossible not to have some sort of prejudice (for instance, the choice of arguments, how to present them and the choice of linguistic terms already constitutes an ideological choice). What really matters is to recognize them, bring them out and manage them, not to avoid them [59]. As for the possibility for the information to change people's behavior, social psychology and its studies [60, 61, 62, 63] have already demonstrated how influence of information does not suffice to modify people's mindset, which tends to understand information in the way they have already become used to thinking.

This said, however, there remains the necessity for making available to the community increasingly clear scientific knowledge, although it does not mean that this information can change the mindset of smokers.

5.1.4. Approach Focused on Emotional Emphasis of Risks

This is neither an objective nor an impartial information approach; rather, it uses emotional communications to threaten listeners about the risk of contracting a disease. Such intervention aims to arouse feelings of fear and concern to provoke a change in the behavior of the receiving subject. The advertising of the '80s contains well-known examples, in which somatic changes induced by drugs were shown, or images of damaged lungs on the cover of some cigarette packs, as well as images of a smoking skeleton, a burned chest, a blackened lung, and pictures of traffic accidents and crushed cars.

The requirement is to provoke reactions in the smoking individual based on the fear of falling ill and the same requirement lies at the basis of many speeches given by teachers, educators, psychologists and doctors who talk to students, as well as parents in conversing with their children. Such an approach can develop emotional reactions that lead listeners to deny the content presented. Moreover, there would be a potential change due to fear and not through a path of awareness; so that once the fear is gone, the risk behavior could come back. Many studies agree with the idea that conditions of fear do not facilitate a real change in behavior [64, 65, 66]. The imposition of a change through threat, as well as the imposition of a healthy behavior, is based on an asymmetrical educational, top-down pattern that is very similar to the doctor-patient pattern. This pattern can be very simple and coherent for those who are used to it but, on the other hand, it turns out to be useless for individuals who do not identify themselves in such a relationship. What's more, to change because someone told you so seldom leads to a personally gained change and eventually, various researches have highlighted the boomerang effect, which involves provoking the change that one was trying to avoid. These paradoxical effects occur because some sort of allure is generated at the same time that the behavior is being outlawed. That is what happens in the school environment when an operator, in an attempt to discourage the consumption, mentions all of the aftereffects of a certain substance, triggering curiosity in the students. This effect is also called reactance [67, 68, 69, 70].

5.1.5. Peer Education Strategy

Peer education is a strategy based on the relationship of mutual influence between people who belong to the same benchmark group [71]. This mutual influence can occur in a formal or an informal way. The term peer has different meanings and can be applied to age, experience, social conditions, school organization, etc. [72, 73] The "peer education" working model has been validated by several studies and research, mostly in the social environment. All of these works [74, 75, 76, 77] demonstrated that individuals are able to change their way of thinking in response to processes of social influence which occur within the peer group or in a significant way of life; peers manage to be more persuasive than adults by using a shared heritage of linguistics and values [78], leading in many cases to an effective change in others' behavior. Several school institutions have noticed the importance of the kind of communication in learning pathways; adult-child interaction could be more stressful to the child than interaction with a peer [79, 80]. From this point, various educational models and applications [81, 82] were developed and, so far, results have been mostly considered favorable. Nevertheless, the necessity to improve the assessment system of interventions suggested by Harden et al. [82] still exists, and especially to plan interventions aimed at triggering competences of participants and not only with information materials. This strategy has frequently been used as an instrument to persuade peers on some themes presented by other peers. The term education has often been used as a synonym of instruction, confining the strategy of peer education among methodologies linked to the transmission of knowledge.

5.2. Interventions Aimed at Developing Skills

Such preparation points for developing the mindset of individuals in the direction of health focus especially on those mindset competences which allow the anticipation of risk situations and management of all the problematic aspects regarding the consumption. It is not about introducing a different behavior but about creating the conditions necessary to develop a new way of seeing things, a new way of interpreting consumption and health.

5.2.1. Self-Empowerment and Community Empowerment Approach

Barbara Solomon introduced the term "empowerment" in the United States in the mid-1970s. It derives from the propulsive and emancipative power of several international organizations aimed at preserving civil rights. Later on, it spread to several other contexts including the political, civil, commercial and above all psychosocial contexts.

There are different ways to interpret this concept; in some cases it seems to be an empty and less concrete slogan. Indeed, there are few empowerment interventions *tout court* (from design to evaluation), just because of the remarkable number of meanings that can be conferred to the concept itself. The idea that it is a development process of one's own abilities toward a greater self-determination of choices regarding the way of organizing one's own life is nevertheless shared. Empowerment, unlike those medical and deficit grounded perspectives, consists in the activation of discovery processes and development of competences and individual, as well as group resources. Referring to the promotion of health, empowerment is considered by the World Health Organization as "that process thanks to which people gain a greater control on their own decisions and initiatives regarding their own health" [83].

Empowerment is divided into individual empowerment and community empowerment. The first refers to the process by which the individual's competences of taking decisions for his/her own life are increased. The second aims to improve the health acting at a socioeconomic and environmental level within the community. Recognizing the correlation between personal health and social contexts means not limiting ourselves to increasing the abilities and the control of individual but instead activating processes of empowerment among the whole community.

The development of many self-determination competences is also named the "culture of independence" in several school contexts, to stress the fact that it is more a cultural attitude than an operative change [84]. Typically, in schools the processes of empowerment are intended for school staff, students and their parents. In many cases social organizations which deal with the promotion of health within the school context and outside are involved. Within the concept of empowerment, all of these subjects participate to the activation of a helix process in which also the slightest contribution of one of these roles can engage other individuals, who will in turn provide contributions [85]. According to this preparation, the process itself announces great transformations in the mindsets of the aforementioned protagonists [86].

We can find another practical example in the studies of the Joint Committee on National Health Education Standards [87, 88], a delegation of American organizations which deals with health promotion. This study describes effective tools for reasoning through standards, competences, in terms of health, be it personal, familiar and collective.

1) Students will comprehend concepts related to health promotion and disease prevention to enhance health.
2) Students will analyze the influence of family, peers, culture, media, technology, and other factors on health behaviors.
3) Students will demonstrate the ability to access valid information, products, and services to enhance health.
4) Students will demonstrate the ability to use interpersonal communication skills to enhance health and avoid or reduce health risks.
5) Students will demonstrate the ability to use decision-making skills to enhance health.
6) Students will demonstrate the ability to use goal-setting skills to enhance health.
7) Students will demonstrate the ability to practice health-enhancing behaviors and avoid or reduce health risks.
8) Students will demonstrate the ability to advocate for personal, family, and community health [87, 88].

The aforementioned approach leads away from the transmission of information and modification of individual conduct-oriented approaches because it describes the need for developing general competences aimed toward the building of a *tout court* healthy lifestyle. In concrete terms, it goes from the action of "doing" to the action of "knowing how to do" and, mostly, to the action of "knowing how to think".

Another applicative example of this approach is the well-known *Life Skill Education* program, which derives directly from the proposal of the World Health Organization [89].

Life skills comprise abilities for adaptive and positive behavior, which enable individuals to deal effectively with the demands and challenges of everyday life.

As has been noted, they concern general competences, linked more to life than to a specific contest. There can also be some differences depending on cultural context; however, the World Health Organization pinpoints the following competences oriented to the enhancement of the welfare of adolescents and young people:

- Decision making
- Problem solving
- Creative thinking
- Critical thinking
- Effective communication
- Interpersonal relationship skills
- Self-awareness
- Empathy
- Coping with emotions
- Coping with stress

Decision-making helps us to deal constructively with decisions about our lives. This can have consequences for health if young people actively make decisions about their actions in relation to health by assessing the different options, and what effects different decisions may have.

Problem solving enables us to deal constructively with problems in our lives. Significant problems that are left unresolved can cause mental stress and give rise to accompanying physical strain.

Creative thinking contributes to both decision-making and problem solving by enabling us to explore the available alternatives and various consequences of our actions or non-action. It helps us to look beyond our direct experience, and even if no problem is identified, or no decision is to be made, creative thinking can help us to respond adaptively and with flexibility to the situations of our daily lives.

Critical thinking is an ability to analyze information and experiences in an objective manner. Critical thinking can contribute to health by helping us to recognize and assess the factors that influence attitudes and behavior, such as values, peer pressure, and the media.

Effective communication means that we are able to express ourselves, both verbally and non-verbally, in ways that are appropriate to our cultures and situations. This means being able to express opinions and desires, but also needs and fears. In addition, it may mean being able to ask for advice and help in a time of need.

Interpersonal relationship skills help us to relate in positive ways with the people we interact with. This may mean being able to make and keep friendly relationships, which can be of great importance to our mental and social well-being. It may mean keeping good relations with family members, which are an important source of social support. It may also mean being able to end relationships constructively.

Self-awareness includes our recognition of ourselves, of our character, and of our strengths and weaknesses, desires and dislikes. Developing self-awareness can help us to recognize when we are stressed or feel under pressure. It is also often a prerequisite for effective communication and interpersonal relations, as well as for developing empathy for others.

Empathy is the ability to imagine what life is like for another person, even in a situation that we may not be familiar with. Empathy can help us to understand and accept others who may be very different from ourselves, which can improve social interactions, for example, in situations of ethnic or cultural diversity. Empathy can also help to encourage nurturing behavior toward people in need of care and assistance, or tolerance, as is the case with AIDS sufferers, or people with mental disorders, who may be stigmatized and ostracized by the very people they depend upon for support.

Coping with emotions involves recognizing emotions in ourselves and others, being aware of how emotions influence behavior, and being able to respond to emotions appropriately. Intense emotions, like anger or sorrow, can have negative effects on our health if we do not react appropriately.

Coping with stress is about recognizing the sources of stress in our lives, recognizing how these affect us, and acting in ways that help to control our levels of stress. This may mean that we take action to reduce the sources of stress; for example, by making changes to our physical environment or lifestyle. Or it may mean learning how to relax, so that tensions created by unavoidable stress do not give rise to health problems [89].

5.2.2. Empowered Peer Education Strategy

This kind of strategy represents the evolution of the traditional peer education, taking, however, a significant distance from the latter, firstly by dropping out any informative purpose and secondly by avoiding the notion that peers learn the same ideas as adults. The activities carried out in this approach are different for each student involved, be it a peer tutor or a tutee. As regards peer students, their role is to facilitate the involved students to express their ideas and to promote their participation, by means of discussion. More specifically, their aim is to elaborate certain ideas and then to develop some useful skills to enhance health. Such a role, however, requires some skills to develop it into a training course for the peer tutor. In this regard, the peer education approach is developed by means of processes and acts of empowerment and self-consciousness [90]. Therefore, the ultimate target is not the mere exchange of information on health; instead, it is to develop some macro skills incidental to the aspects of expertise and know-how. This mindset approach appears to be very appropriate for the school environment, if everyone is involved in it [91, 92].

6. Method Indications to Promoting Health

6.1. From the Change in Behavior to the Development of Skills

For several reasons, including the will of adults to protect minors, intervention against tobacco addiction has for a long time been an approach merely aimed at changing the behavior of others. Information activities about the aftereffects of diseases, attempts to emotionally affect students, the prohibition of potentially dangerous consumptions and encounters, are all examples of this kind of approach. Scientific research has highlighted that behavior is always influenced by a certain way of thinking and, even if one manages to modify it, such a modification does not necessarily lead to a change in the general way of thinking. That said, if an individual has a risk propensity, he or she would find many ways to put him or herself in danger, even if a specific risky behavior is prevented. If an individual has a dangerous driving style in riding the motor scooter, imposing a ban would be worthless, since the possibilities of endangering one's life or conducting a risky behavior are multiple.

Nowadays, given the complexity of the health process, also referring to parameters of the World Health Organization, the overview of the individual and his tendency to conduct a healthy or risky behavior is highlighted. Much importance is given to the mindset and its influence on behavior; therefore an intervention in this area is considered essential. Consequently, it causes a different approach to health, a "daily training to the health reasoning" which requires specific competences aimed at promoting this view of life.

6.2. From Identification of the Causes of Consumption to the Research of Intentions

Traditionally, interventions against tobacco addiction have been subjected to the influence of the medical model and of commonsense. The first one oriented the knowledge about smoking to a permanent research of the cause-effect correlation, which led to the assumption that there is an effective cause at the basis of consumption and that this cause needs to be removed. In this way, reductionist models of intervention were established which focused on the removal of the cause rather than on its comprehension. Implicitly, the complex act of smoking has been identified with the underlying biochemical mechanism. Such aspects as the significance the adolescent gives to the act of smoking, the sense that action has for him and his group and the meaning attributed to the act of smoking by family members have been neglected.

In this sense, health is intended not merely as a condition of health or disease but, instead, a greater emphasis is given to its procedures. The focus now is on the significance of the condition of disease within a healthy way of life. Moreover, the comprehension of the reason why an individual chooses to smoke can no longer be separated from the aftereffects individuals aim to reach, be it a physical gratification or, especially, a psychological gratification. The desire of smoking is often linked to the wish to try what is considered by a certain group of people to be an important, pleasant or necessary experience.

6.3. From the Individual Approach to the Analysis of Territorial and School Context

As we have seen, the consumption of tobacco among young individuals is influenced by peers and by the group dynamics to which one belongs.

To understand such a connection, analysis has to take into account the meanings (ideas, beliefs, values) attributed to the act of smoking in the context of belonging and one of which of these meanings is used by the subject to integrate this act into his way of being. Studies on the context of belonging highlight what can foster the act of smoking and what can hinder it; in this logic health is seen as a process involving the major context in which the individual lives and with which he or she interacts. For this reason, health-enhancing activities need to be carried out at a level of individual knowledge as well as by creating reference models shared with the reference environment [89, 93]. In school, the class group represents the reference environment; hence, the fear of "yellow teeth" or "blemished skin" can lead students to change their minds more than the fear of contracting diseases. The meanings given to the act of smoking are attributed from individuals depending on their needs, whether they are psychological, social or relational needs [94].

REFERENCES

[1] Iudici A., & Faccio, E. (2013). The conflict at school: clinical implications and mediation interventions in *Procedia- Social Behavioral Sciences*, vol. 89, p. 901-905.

[2] Council Directive 89/622/EEC of 13 November 1989 on the approximation of the laws, regulations and administrative provisions of the Member States concerning the labeling of tobacco products.

[3] Council Directive 90/239/EEC of 17 May 1990 on the approximation of the laws, regulations and administrative provisions of the Member States concerning the maximum tar yield of cigarettes

[4] Bates, C., McNeil, A., Jarvis, M., & Gray, N. (1999). The future of tobacco product regulation and labeling in Europe: implications for the forthcoming European Union directive. *Tobacco control*, vol. 8, p. 225-135.

[5] Council Directive 92/41/EEC of 15 May 1992: Amending Directive 89/622/EEC on the Approximation of the Laws, Regulations and Administrative Provisions of the Member States Concerning the Labeling of Tobacco Products.

[6] Council Directive 95/59/EC of 27 November 1995 on taxes other than turnover taxes which affect the consumption of manufactured tobacco.

[7] Council Directive 1999/81/EC of 29 July 1999 amending Directive 92/79/EEC on the approximation of taxes on cigarettes, Directive

92/80/EEC on the approximation of taxes on manufactured tobacco other than cigarettes and Directive 95/59/EC on taxes other than turnover taxes which affect the consumption of manufactured tobacco (7).

[8] Gallus, S., Schiaffino, A., La Vecchia, C., Townsend, J., & Fernandez, E. (2006). Price and Cigarette consumption in Europe. *Tobacco Control*, 15, 2, p. 114-119.

[9] Rossi, S., Pizzi, E., Mastrobattista, L., Spoletini, R., Carosi, G., & Pacifici, R. (2006). *Politica di controllo del tabagismo: Aumento dei Prezzi.* Istituto Superiore di Sanità, OSSFAD.

[10] Directive 2001/37/EC of the European Parliament and of the Council of 5 June 2001 on the approximation of the laws, regulations and administrative provisions of the Member States concerning the manufacture, presentation and sale of tobacco products.

[11] World Health Organization (2013). *WHO Report on the Global Tobacco Epidemic: Enforcing bans on tobacco advertising, promotion and sponsorship.* Avaible at http://www.who.int/tobacco/global_report/2013/en/

[12] Fiore, M.C., Jaén, C.R.; Baker, T.B., Bailey, W.C., Benowitz, N.L.; Curry, S.J., Dorfman, S.F., Froelicher, E.S., Goldstein, M.G., & Healton, C.G.(2008) *Treating Tobacco Use and Dependence: Update.* U.S. Department of Health and Human Services, Public Health Service: Rockville.

[13] Sandstrom P. (2003) *Evaluation of the European Network on Young People and Tobacco* (ENYPAT) 1997–2002. Helsinki, Finland: National Public Health Institute.

[14] Jha, P., Jacob, B., Gajalakshmi, V., Gupta, P.C., Dhingra, N., Kumar, R., Sinha, D.N., Dikshit, R.P., Parida, D.K., Kamadod, R., Boreham, J., & Peto, R. (2008), RGI-CGHR Investigators: A nationally representative case-control study of smoking and death in India. *N. Engl. J. Med.*, *358*, 1137-1147.

[15] Lopez, A.D., Mathers, C.D., Ezzati, M., Jamison, D.T., & Murray, C.J. Global and regional burden of disease and risk factors (2001) Systematic analysis of population health data. *Lancet* 2006, *367*, 1747–1757.

[16] Al Ghobain, M.O., Al Moamary, M.S., Al Shehri, S.N., & Al-Hajjaj, M.S. (2011). Prevalence and characteristics of cigarette smoking among 16 to 18 years old boys and girls in Saudi Arabia. *Ann.Thorac. Med,* 6, p. 137–140.

[17] Palipudi, K.M., Gupta, P.C., Sinha, D.N., Andes, L.J., Asma, S., & McAfee, T. (2012). GATS Collaborative Group. Social determinants of health and tobacco use in thirteen low and middle income countries: Evidence from Global Adult Tobacco Survey. *PLoS ONE* 2012, *7*, doi:10.1371/journal. pone.0033466.

[18] World Health Organization (WHO) (2011). *WHO Report on the Global Tobacco Epidemic*. Geneva: World Health Organization.

[19] Conner, M., Grogan, S., Lawton, R., & Armitage C. (2013) Study protocol: A cluster randomised controlled trial of implementation intentions to reduce smoking initiation in adolescents. *Bmc Public Health* Volume: 13 Article Number: 54.

[20] Jha, P., Ranson, M.K., Nguyen, S.N., & Yach, D.P. (2002) Estimates of global and regional smoking prevalence in 1995, by ageand sex. *Amer. J. Pub. Health*, *6*, p. 1002–1006.

[21] World Health Organization: *WHO Framework Convention on Tobacco Control (2003)* Geneva: World Health Organization.

[22] Cogliano, V., Straif, K., Baan, R., Grosse, Y., Secretan, B., & El Ghissassi, F. (2004). Smokeless tobacco and tobacco-related nitrosamines. *Lancet Oncol*; 5:708.

[23] Brook, J.S., & Brook, D.W. (2004) Zhang, C.; Cohen, P. Tobacco use and health in young adulthood. *J. Genet. Psychol.* 165, p. 310–323.

[24] Becklake, M.R., Ghezzo, H., & Ernst, P. (2005). Childhood predictors of smoking in adolescence: A follow up study of Montreal schoolchildren. *CMAJ*, *173*, p. 377–379.

[25] Lasser, K., Boyd, J. W., Woolhandler, S., Himmelstein, D. U., McCormick, D., & Bor, D. H. (2000). Smoking and mental Illness: a population based prevalence study. *The Journal of the American Medical Association,* Vol. 284, 20, p. 2606-2610.

[26] Dani, J. A., & Harris, A. R. (2005). Nicotine addiction and comorbidity with alcohol abuse and mental illness. *Nature neuroscience*, Vol. 8, 11, 1465-1470.

[27] De Leon, J., & Diaz, F.J. (2005). A meta-analysis of worldwide studies demonstrates an association between schizophrenia and tobacco smoking behaviors. *Schizophrenia Research*, 76, p. 135-157.

[28] Simon Morton, B., Crump, A.D., Haynie, D.L., & Taylor, K.E. (1999). Pshicological, school and parents factors associated with smoking in university students. *Prev Med*, 28, p. 138-148.

[29] Button, T.M.M., Thapar, A., & McGuffin, P. (2005). Relationship between antisocial behaviour, attention-deficit hyperactivity disorder

and maternal prenatal smoking. *British Journal of Psychiatry*, 187, p. 155–160

[30] Wakschlag, L.S., Pickett, K.E., Cook, E., Benowitz, N.L., & Leventhal, B.L. (2002). Maternal smoking during pregnancy and severe antisocial behavior in offspring: A review. *American Journal of Public Health*, 92, p. 966-974.

[31] Word Health Organization (1986). *Ottawa Charter Health Promotion*. Regional Office For Europe.

[32] The European convention. *European-convention*. eu.int. Retrieved 2014-04-01. http://european-convention.eu.int/EN/bienvenue/bienvenue2352.html? lang =EN.

[33] Paavola M., Vartiainen P., & Puska, P. (1996). Predicting adult smoking: The influence of smoking during adolescent and smoking among friends and family. *Health Educ Res*, 11: 309-315.

[34] Difranza, J.R., Rigotti, N.A., McNeill, A.D., Ockene, J.K., Savageau, J.A., St Cyr, D., & Coleman, M. (2000). Initial symptoms of nicotine dependence in adolescents. *Tob Control*, 9 (3), p. 313-319.

[35] Gollwitzer, P.M., & Sheeran, P. (2006). Implementation intentions and goal achievement: A meta-analysis of effects and processes. *Adv Exp Soc Psychol*, 38, p. 69-119.

[36] Chassing, L., Presson, C., Rose, J., Sherman, S. J., & Prost, J. (2002). Parental smoking cessation and adolescent smoking. *Journal of Pediatric Psychology*, vol. 27, (6), p. 485-496.

[37] Hoeflmayr, D., & Hanewinkel, R. (2008). Do school-based tobacco prevention programmes, pay off? The cost-effectivness of the "smoke-freeclass competition". *Journal of the Royal Institute of Public Health*, 122, p. 34-41.

[38] Stevens, S.L., Colwell, B., Smith, D.W., Robinson, J., & McMillan, C. (2005). An exploration of self-reported negative affect by adolescents as a reason for smoking: implications for tobacco prevention and intervention programs. *Preventive Medicine*, vol. 41 (2), p. 589–596.

[39] Tengs, T.O., Osgood, N.D., & Chen, L.L. (2001). The cost-effectiveness of intensive national school-based anti-tobacco Education: Result from the tobacco policy model. *Preventive Medicine*, Vol. 33, p. 558-570.

[40] Sussman, S., Lichtman, K., Ritt, A., & Pallonen, U.E. (1999) Effects of thirty-four adolescent tobacco use cessation and prevention trials on regular users of tobacco products. *Subst Use Misuse*, 34 (11), p. 1469-1503.

[41] Sussman S. (2002). Effects of sixty six adolescent tobacco use cessation trials and seventeen prospective studies of self-initiated quitting. *Tob Induc Dis*, 1(1): 35-81.

[42] Grimshaw, G.M., & Stanton A. (2006). Tobacco cessation interventions for young people. *Cochrane Database Syst Rev* (4):CD003289.

[43] Gervais, A., O'Loughlin, J., Dugas, E., Eisenberg, M.J., Wellman, R.J., & Difranza, J.R. (2007). A systematic review of randomized controlled trials of youth smoking cessation interventions. *Drogues, santé et société*, 6(1), p. 283-316.

[44] Minary, L., Cambon, L., Martini, H., Wirth, N., Acouetey, D.S., Thouvenot, F., Maire, C., Martinet, Y., Bohadana, A., Zmirou-Navier, D., & Alla, F. (2013). Efficacy of a smoking cessation program in a population of adolescent smokers in vocational schools: a public health evaluative controlled study. *BMC public health*, February, 13: 149. Springer.

[45] Thomas, R. (2002). *School-based Programmes for Preventing Smoking (Cochrane Review)*. The Library. Oxford: Update Software.

[46] Garrison, M.M., Christakis, D.A., Ebel, B.E., Wiehe, S.E., & Rivara, F.P. (2003). Smoking cessation interventions for adolescents: a systematic review. *Am J Prev Med*, 25(4), p. 363-367.

[47] Wiehe, S.E., Garrison, M.M., Christakis, D.A., Ebel, B.E., & Rivara, F.P. (2005). A systematic review of school-based smoking prevention trials with long-term follow-up. *J Adolesc Health*, 36, p. 162-9.

[48] Turchi, G.P., & Della Torre, C. (2007). *Psicologia della salute - dal modello bio-psico-sociale al modello dialogico: generare e gestire processi trasformativi nell'ambito della "salute"*. Roma: Armando.

[49] Burkhart, G. (2003). *Report on selective prevention in the European union and Norway, selective prevention*. European Monitoring Centre for drugs and drugs addiction.

[50] Barattini, B. (1999), "Orientamenti culturali e metodologici sulla prevenzione delle dipendenze", *Animazione sociale*, 3, p. 91-93.

[51] Cohen, P. (1999). Shifting the Main Purposes of Drug Control. *The International Journal of Drug Policy*, 10, p. 223-234; tr. it. "Un mutamento di rotta degli obiettivi principali del controllo sulla droga". *Quaderni di Fuoriluogo*, 7. Editore Forum Droghe, Roma.

[52] Chavis, D.M., De Pietro, G., & Martini, E.R. (1994). Prevenzione del disagio e sviluppo di comunità: concetti di base e strategie operative. *Animazione sociale*, vol. 24 (4), p. 9-20.

[53] Hawkins, J.D., Catalano, R.F. & Arthur, M. (2002). Promoting science-based prevention in communities. *Addictive Behaviors,* 90 (5), p. 1–26.
[54] National Institute on Drug Abuse Research Report (2004). *Cocaine Abuse and Addiction: NIH Publication No. 99-4342*. Printed May Revised November.
[55] Backinger, C.L., Fagan, P., Matthews E., & Grana, R. (2003). Adolescent and young adult tobacco prevention and cessation: current status and future directions. *Tob Control* 2003, 12 (Suppl 4), p. IV46-IV53.
[56] McDonald, P., Colwell, B., Backinger, C.L., Husten, C., & Maule, C.O. (2003). Better practices for youth tobacco cessation: evidence of review panel. *Am J Health Behav* 2003, 27(Suppl 2): p. S144-S158.
[57] Gray, N., Henningfield, J.E., Benowitz, N. L., Connolly, G. N., Dresler, C., Fagerström, K., Jarvis, M. J., & Boyle, P. (2005). Toward a comprehensive long term nicotine policy. *Tobacco Control*, 14, p. 161-165.
[58] Watzlavich, P. (1984). *The Invented Reality: How Do We Know What We Believe We Know? (Contributions to Constructivism)*. New York: Norton.
[59] Gadamer, H.G. (1982). *Truth & method*. New York: Crossroad
[60] Hansen, W.B. (1992). School-based substance abuse prevention: A review of the state of the art in curriculum, 1980–1990. *Health Education Research: Theory and Practice*, 7, 403–430.
[61] Tobler, N., & Stratton, H. (1997). Effectiveness of school-based drug education programs: a meta-analysis of the research. *Journal of Primary Prevention*, 18, (1), p. 71-128.
[62] Tobler, N.S., Roona, M.R., Ochshorn, P., Marshall, D.G., Streke, A.V., & Stackpole, K.M. (2000). School-based adolescent drug preventionprograms: 1998 meta-analysis. *Journal of Primary Prevention*, 20, p. 275-337.
[63] Smith, D.R., L'Abbate, N., & Lorusso, A.(2008). Tobacco smoking among Italian physicians and the role of occupational medicine. *Med Lav*, 99, p. 3-7.
[64] Evans, R.G., & Stoddart, G.L. (1990). Producing health, consuming health care. *Social Science and Medicine,* 31 (12), p. 1347-1363.
[65] Tartarotti, L. (1986). *Droga e prevenzione primaria: prospettive e strategie dell'intervento preventivo scolastico*. Milano: Giuffrè.

[66] Bonino S., & Cattelino E. (a cura di) (2008). *La prevenzione in adolescenza: percorsi psicoeducativi di intervento sul rischio e la salute*. Gardolo: Erikson.

[67] Brehm, J. W. (1966). *A theory of psychological reactance*. New York: Academic Press.

[68] Hyland, M., & Birrell, J. (1979). Government health warnings and the" boomerang" effect. *Psychological Reports,* 44, p. 643-7.

[69] Tartarotti, L. (2010). *Psicologia della salute: un'introduzione*. Milano: Franco Angeli.

[70] Buscema, M. (1986). *Prevenzione e dissuasione*. Torino: EGA.

[71] Starkey, F., Audrey, S., Holliday, J., Moore, J., L., & Campbell, R. (2009). Identifying influential young people to undertake effective peer-led health promotion: the example of A Stop Smoking In Schools Trial (ASSIST). *Health Educ. Res*., 24 (6), p. 977-988. Oxford Univ. Press.

[72] Orme, J, & Starkey, F. (1999). Peer drug education: the way forward? *Health Education*, 1, p. 8–16.

[73] Shiner, M., & Newburn, T. (1997). Definitely, Maybe Not? The Normalisation of Recreational Drug Use amongst Young People. *Sociology* 31(3), p. 511–29.

[74] Damon, W., & Killen, M. (1982). Peer interaction and the process of change in children's moral reasoning. *Merrill-Palmer Quarterly,* 28, p.347-378.

[75] Damon, W. (1984). Peer education: The untapped potential. *Journal of Applied Developmental Psychology,* 5, p. 331-343.

[76] Turner, G. & Sheperd, J. (1999) A method in search of a theory: peer education and health promotion. *Health Education Research*, 14, p. 235–247.

[77] Milburn, K. (1995). A critical review of peer education with young people with special reference to sexual health. *Health Education Research*, 10, p. 407–420.

[78] Valente, T.W., Davis, R.L., (1999). Accelerating the diffusion of innovations using opinion leaders. *The Annals of the American Academy of the Political and Social Sciences*, 566, p. 55-67.

[79] Boda, G. (2001). *Life skills e peer education: strategie per l'efficacia personale e collettiva.* Milano: La Nuova Italia.

[80] Pepe, S. (2004). L'educazione tra pari: una bibliografia ragionata. *Psicologia dell'Educazione e della Formazione*, Gardolo: Erikson, 6, p. 89-107.

[81] Hoffman, B.R., Sussman, S., Unger, J.B., Valente, T.W. (2006). Peer influences on adolescent cigarette smoking: a theoretical review of the literature. *Subs Use Misuse*, 41, p. 103-155.

[82] Harden, A., Weston, R., Oakley, A. (1999). *A review of the effectiveness and appropriateness of peer-delivered health promotion interventions for young people.* London: EPPI-Centre.

[83] World Health Organization (2008). *MPOWER: A Policy Package to Reverse the Tobacco Epidemic*. Geneva: World Health Organization.

[84] Cesarini, G. & Regni, R. (1999). *Autonomia e empowerment. L'educazione e le nuove frontiere dell'organizzazione.* Roma: Armando.

[85] Barksdale-Ladd, M.A. & Thomas, K.F. (1996). The Development of Empowerment in Reading Instruction in Eight Elementary Teachers. *Teaching and Teacher Education*, 12, p. 161-178.

[86] Iudici, A., Rumi, G., Faccio, E., Maiocchi, A., de Aloe, S. (2013) From the clinical findings related to the victimization to the mediation of the conflict. Description of an experience of peer mediation in an Italian school. *European Journal Of Social Behaviour*, vol. V, n. 2, p. 1015-1023.

[87] Joint Committee on National Health Education Standards (1995). *National health education standards: Achieving health literacy.* Atlanta, GA: American Cancer Society.

[88] Joint Commitee on National Health Stand. *National Health Education Standards* (2007). Atlanta, GA: American Cancer Society.

[89] WHO (1994) *Life skills education for children and adolescents in schools. Pt. 1, Introduction to life skills for psychosocial competence. Pt. 2, Guidelines to facilitate the development and implementation of life skills programmes.* Geneva : World Health Organization

[90] Pearson, M., Chilton, R., Woods, H.B, Wyatt K., Ford, T., Abraham, C. & Anderson, R. (2012) Implementing health promotion in schools: protocol for a realist systematic review of research and experience in the United Kingdom (UK). *Systematic Reviews*, 1, 48.

[91] Deschesnes, M., Martin, C., & Hill, A.J. (2003). Comprehensive approaches to school promotion: how to achieve broader implementation? *Health Promotion International*, 18, 4, p. 387-396.

[92] Weare, K. (1995). The contribution of education to health promotion. In: Bunton, R., & Macdonald, G. *Health promotion: disciplines and diversity.* London (UK): Routledge.

[93] Iudici, A. (2014) Skills-Lab Project. Promoting the integration of diversity as a culture of participation. Community relief, economic, social, clinical and health. *Procedia- Social Behavioral Sciences*, vol. 116, p. 3636-40.

[94] Iudici, A. Faccio, E., Salvini, A.(2013). A new way to oppose the consumption of drugs: the toxicophilia. New methodological tools for the promotion of health and for the clinic. *European Journal Of Social Behaviour*, vol. V, n. 2, pag. 985- 994.

Chapter 5

DEVIANCE AND SCHOOL: HISTORICAL REFERENCES, CONCEPTS AND METHODS OF INTERVENTION

1. INTRODUCTION

As is known, school is a place for knowledge and a context of social relations that can sometimes be conflicting. These conflicts may involve students, school institutions and in some cases parents and teachers. Conflicting situations need to be managed; otherwise, they may have a negative effect on coexistence in school and on academic performance. Scientific literature has long highlighted data on these consequences; for example, a conflicting environment can lead to poor attendance, skipping classes, and quitting school [1, 2, 3]. Moreover, a conflicting environment at school may result in situations of personal discomfort, refusal, self-exclusion, threats, and alienation, affecting the quality and effectiveness of the learning process [4, 5]. Dropouts and conflicts are not always the result of the malfunction of the school but they may have a meaning in a broader context that is the social context of which the school is part. For instance, an aggressive and provocative behavior in school is often due to the way the person deals with problems outside the school [6].

In many cases, younger people tend to identify themselves with those who have antisocial behavior, even if the deviant conduct is identified as a juvenile deviance. Authorities do not necessarily punish such deviant acts because many of the violations committed are not even identified; nonetheless, the problematic behavior may be at risk of becoming a deviant behavior and of strengthening itself both within the school context and outside of it. Therefore, helping the school to manage such deviant situations appears even more important. The general definition of the term deviance is a set of behaviors that break the complexity of values, regulations and principles that, at a given historical moment and in a given social context, are valid and fundamental in the culture of the dominant social group [7]. To achieve this goal, it is necessary to adopt specific methodologies and tools to involve several public institutions (courthouses, municipalities, provinces, regions, and universities) and private organizations (associations and social cooperatives). Of course, the institution of the school takes a key position in this context, due to the opportunity to identify the development path of students and therefore of future citizens.

2. Measures Against Juvenile Deviance: Research Contributions and Clinical Implications

Scientific literature shows that deviance increases in the period between 12 and 14 years [8], reaching its height between 17 and 19 years and slowly decreasing afterwards [9]. In many studies, reference is made to the risky behaviors [10]; in other studies, to the antisocial behavior [11] and in yet others, to the deviant action [12] and criminal behavior [13]. There are many studies which attribute deviant behavior to the family; in many cases, children tend to repeat their parents' hard attitude [14], and in other cases children learn the manners used by their parents during conflicts [15]. In yet other cases children don't receive any incentive to behave legally and they are left free to act the way they want to in their youth [16, 17]. All this leads children to come into contact with territory without any ability to filter the events, to establish important relations with friends and to get to know their friends' families and values. The fact that children don't spend time with their families and, above all, don't share their experiences with them can lead them to agree with stimuli coming from their peer group and to identifying themselves with those stimuli. Such experience, if not shared with the adults around them, may be an experience as an end in itself, rather than as a means for personal growth. The act of smoking and the consumption of alcohol are widespread experiences among young people and they may become permanent habits [18].

Several authors agree in saying that this is a fundamental phase for children because in this period prerequisites for building one's own identity are established, whether they are deviant or not. By contrast, the ability of parents to play a role in supervising their kids' experiences often leads to a reduction of deviant experiences [19]. Of course, it is not always easy to distinguish between problematic behavior and deviance [20]; however, we think that one of the requirements of school is to equip itself with tools to understand how to hinder the development of deviant behavior before it becomes effective. To meet this need, let us now highlight the patterns and theories from which it becomes possible to schedule a contrasting intervention to tackle deviance at school.

3. Approaches to Juvenile Deviance

To understand juvenile deviance is a very difficult process; to intervene to hinder it is a challenge. There are different approaches to this theme and different operating practices have developed. For the purpose of this publication, we will distinguish two macro approaches, both useful for school intervention. The first one concerns etiological theories of deviance, which aim to identify the main causes of the deviant behavior, whether they are bio-medical, psychological or sociological. The second one concerns theories that see deviance as a social construction process and therefore aim to comprehend how the deviant act is produced.

3.1. Etiological Theories of Deviance

The first researchers to deal with deviance were interested in searching deviant behavior for some "sure" and objective factors. We are referring to constitutional theories and psychiatric studies.

The former refer to the so-called classical school and to the positivist criminology [21, 22]. Cesare Lombroso, an Italian doctor, is certainly among the most influential exponents of this approach. Practicing the lobotomy of a criminal's skull, he individuated a brain cleft, typical of lower animals. He deduced that this calf was a congenital morphological anomaly, which could explain the difference between a criminal and a reasonable person. He therefore coined the term "born criminal", to describe the notion that the criminal person is a primitive being with uncontrollable ferocious instincts [23]. Such observations have been developed by his pupil, Enrico Ferri, who identified physical (geography, ethnic group, climate), anthropological (age, sex, psyche) and social (customs, religion, economy) aspects as the main factors of delinquency. Raffaele Garofalo [24], another scholar of this movement, individuated a set of natural and environmental causes underlying the criminal behavior, expressing the existence of physical and psychological anomalies among the individuals of the so-called "lower races". This approach postulated the existence of a close correlation between the deviant conduct and some physical features or chromosomal abnormalities. Consistent with this idea is the hypothesis that the presence of a neurological or glandular deficit can be considered at the basis of socially reproachable behavior.

Another line of study proposed to consider the criminal act as a result of some specific psychopathological conditions. The hypothesis that criminal behavior would be displayed in individuals with psychiatric pathology was developed. Various studies [see 12] have ratified that there is only a marginal link between deviant behavior and insanity. The latter, although a symbolic and dramatized aspect of the diversity, is nothing but a marginal part of deviant behaviors, which cannot be conceptually integrated into mental illness. Nevertheless, the medical-psychiatric orientation will progressively take hold and spread among some deviant behaviors totally beyond medical competence. At this point, the problem is to understand why the sanitarian world claimed such knowledge and competences within the context of social control. The spread of a conception of the world governed by mechanical and universal, physical and biological, and social and economic laws beyond the control of individuals, leads to the certainty that human behavior could be reduced to the inflexible law of natural determinism, whether it is biopsychological or social. Such an assumption allowed explaining deviance by means of causal mechanisms for a long time. The claimed precondition of laying the foundations of the behavioral and ethical-social normality criteria on biological knowledge explains why public authorities resorted to the practices of criminal anthropology, forensic medicine and psychiatry, allowing them to take over the social and legal sphere with their criteria of normality and pathology [25].

These studies made a big methodological mistake, which is studying the renowned crime (and not the hidden one) without a control group, producing the common idea that insanity and criminality are two inseparable aspects [12]. Although today common feeling still considers this idea as true, most crimes are committed by non-disabled individuals.

Caplan [26]'s studies suggest another medical approach, which defines intervention toward criminal behavior as prevention. The author identifies three different types of prevention; the first is primary prevention, aimed to eliminate criminogenic factors in the physical and social environment, by means of educational, political, social and urban interventions. Secondary prevention is aimed toward the early individuation of potential criminals, especially among young people. Tertiary prevention takes place after a crime is committed and aims to prevent the recurrence of it. Other types of prevention focus on areas of intervention and on the people to whom the intervention is addressed. For instance, the term social prevention is widely used, partly matching with primary prevention, but using methodologies belonging to social sciences [27, 28, 29].

In scientific literature, situational prevention is aimed at physically preventing the accomplishment of crimes. Another type of individual prevention based on predictive researches of human behavior is oriented toward children and adolescents with potential "crime-risk" [30].

In addition to the medical approach, in scientific literature some sociological deviance explanations are also available. At first, these explanations were influenced by references of social Darwinism; later, the attention was drawn to social organization, due also to the studies of some important social theorists such as Durkheim, Parsons and Merton.

3.1.1. Durkheim's Anomie Theory

The French sociologist has made very important contributions to social sciences; to him we owe the difference between social and natural areas, as well as the importance of their normative criteria. To him we also owe the idea that crime has a role within society; for instance, the role to define what is allowed and what is not, to allow non-deviant individuals to consider themselves as "fair", to induce reflection on how at certain times a behavior is considered to be deviant, to enhance the presence of reassuring social roles such as the judge, or the attorney, whose existence is due to the existence of crime and to ensure an efficient and safe system. To the author, deviance is an element of disunity that ends up having a cohesion impact due to the control system that it produces.

According to anomie theory, deviance is established when a separation between cultural structure and social structure takes place. The first one includes the set of ambitions and ideas with which the reference society identifies; the latter includes the interactive rules used by people to relate. When cultural targets, which the society is striving toward, are different from the social-relational possibilities, then some rules of civil coexistence lose their meaning and people tend not to respect them anymore. The lack, loss or dearth of such rules is called anomie and it is considered to be the cause of deviance [31]. Afterwards, thanks to Durkheim's studies on suicide [32], he adopted the term anomie to refer to the morally deregulated condition due to which individuals have little control over their behavior. However, the subject's lack of intention and his behavior are due to the completely social organization. Later, anomie theory was reviewed by different currents of thoughts, different disciplines and by authors such as Sutherland, Parson and Merton.

3.1.2. T. Parson's Structural-Functionalism

Contrary to Durkheim, Talcott Parson highlights in his studies the active role of the subject. According to the author, human behavior has elements of voluntariness and does not directly depend on a structural conflict between cultural and social aspects, nor between classes or different class interests. Deviance (role-expectation) is considered the effect of the subject's incapacity to integrate in the set of values and expectations of society, in relation to his socialization and to the set of biographic, personal and environmental elements [33]. According to Parson, identification, introjections and internalization of the regulatory system, including goals, values and models of behavior, did not suffice or were disturbed. In this sense, deviancy is depicted as a failure to adapt to the social reality; indeed, the problem is to motivate deviants to follow the rules of social organization. This entails a set of different interventions to correct, cure or re-socialize individuals. Less attention is given to repressive or custody interventions, typical of the preceding approach.

3.1.3. Differential Association Theory

This theory, formulated by Sutherland and formalized with the collaboration of Cressey [34], assumes that the deviant behavior is socially learned. According to the authors, deviance is produced by the learning of a set of values, regulations and attitudes within the society but in contrast with the dominating culture. To some extent deviance is a self-produced process of the social context, applied thanks to individuals or groups who give positive meanings to deviant behaviors and offer means for their realization [35]. According to De Leo and Patrizi [12], differential association theory has an explanatory importance for the subject in the evolutionary age who is building his own normative dimension compared with the conduct to be adopted. In fact, even though it does not explain the onset of deviance, it is a first theoretical threshold that sees deviance as a learning process in time and in relations. Another critical aspect of this approach is that it does not explain how individuals from the same social context and with the same established relations do not have the same deviant reactions.

3.1.4. Merton's Anomie Theory

Merton's theory partly repeats Durkheim's anomie theory; he asserts that there are some goals within the society, in the form of desires and purposes, legitimated by the social context itself. Not all individuals can achieve all of these aims; consequently, the phenomena of disparity and social disintegration may arise. However, a cultural goal that is constantly emphasized triggers the possibility that the goal itself can only be achieved through the violation of some of the institutional regulations. Such conditions lead to ignoring regulations (anomie) from which deviant behaviors are produced, due to a disharmony between existential aims offered by the social culture and the legitimate means to achieve them. To some extent the author sees deviance as an "average" reaction to pressures from society in a pathological way. Moreover, not considering the moral aspects, the scholar also identifies in the deviance a creative and innovative factor, essential to social change.

Merton's studies [37, 38] had a significant impact on the field of social sciences and opened the doors for new possibilities of research and knowledge. First, there is the certainty that studies on deviance are not necessarily related to legal issues; it is very useful to study social, psychological and relational processes involved in this phenomenon even if there is no crime committed. This is a very important feature for scholars of deviance, as it has allowed the overcoming of the methodological boundary thus far implemented, which has restricted scientific study only to those subjects intercepted by law. Therefore, such studies allow for studying deviance also by means of how the phenomenon materializes through different perspectives. Moreover, according to Merton, it needs to identify deviations in a broader way, not only through the categories of "crime" and "disease", to understand the different manifestations of the same deviations. This is a very important contribution also to other disciplines, as it focuses on the comprehension of the different faces of a phenomenon instead of explaining it through self-serving prototypes of categories.

Due to Merton [39], the merger between normative deviance and ethical-moral aspects, a very important concept, has also been overcome. Among the critical aspects of Merton's approach there is the difficulty of explaining those deviant acts which are not due to the pursuit of social and cultural desires. Moreover, to aim at the same cultural goals there must be an adequate socialization, but in many deviants this is not so. Furthermore, when referring to cultural goals, Merton runs the risk of making them objective and out-of-the-context elements; hence, there is the risk of not taking into account the relativity aspect of the goals depending on the reference system.

3.1.5. Cohen's Subculture Theory

This approach is inspired by studies mainly involving young individuals. Taking into account some of Merton's observations, the authors of this approach have long studied youth gangs, neighborhood activities, and communities of adolescents, highlighting the presence of a criminal youth subculture, with a set of regulations, values and ideas acquired by young people in contrast to the dominating culture. According to Cohen [40], most young people are in search of a specific social status but not everyone can reach it by means of the same opportunities, especially lower-class children who lack material and symbolic benefits. Such frustration may lead to various types of adaptation to the values of the middle classes, which, in some cases, can lead to an establishment of a new set of regulations or to the legitimating of behaviors in opposition to the middle classes. Such regulations take on an alternative cultural form, called subculture delinquency. Taking into account some of Merton's suggestions, the author asserts that tensions produced by social disintegration produce a strong social unease in many young individuals of the lower classes, who may believe that the best solution to such a problem is to participate in subculture delinquency.

Cloword and Ohlin [41] asserted that there are many ways in which young people manage to achieve their ambitions (differential opportunity theory). In urban areas inhabited by lower classes, where there are few opportunities for personal growth, other opportunities take place; however, even these opportunities offer limited access. Hence, social position defines the competence of using both legitimate and illegal roads to success. Such a hypothesis is supported by the fact that, as an individual makes his way into the criminal business, he is given the necessary means to start his own business. In this case, deviance is an "apprenticeship structure" on which to train in order to find a social integration [35].

Deviant subculture theory's weakness, as Lemert states [42], is in its indiscriminate use and the concept of "culture", which ends up becoming an empirical data that is considered the cause of the phenomenon, or often not even related to it. It is a matter of fact that the notion of deviant subculture can be easily misused and misinterpreted by the non-expert, turning into a verbal *passé partout*, as it is the concept of the subconscious. These words are easily misused because of their easy interpretation. The concept of "culture" is used (and misused) in common meaning to explain some social phenomena; however, the way this word is simplified means it cannot describe such a complex phenomenon.

3.1.6. Bandura's Social Learning Theory

Bandura distances himself from the idea that people change their behavior depending on prices and punishments; instead, he highlights the learning process (modeling) according to which a person tends to modify his behavior after the observation of another person. Such a process does not require direct contact between the two people but can be activated through indirect experiences. According to the author [43, 44], this learning process, also known as vicarious, is based on identification between the modeler and the modeled. Among the most influential properties on the production of a modeling situation, there are similarity of performances, similarity of personal characteristics among observer and model, multiplicity and variety of models and finally, the proficiency of the model [45].

According to Bandura, then, deviance is the effect of a modeling process as regards to patterns within our society, which are appropriated by specific cognitive mechanisms. According to all of the aforementioned theories, deviance is a given social problem, whether its causes are social, cultural, psychological or genetic.

3.2. Processual Theories of Deviance

In opposition to the aforementioned theories, an approach has been developed that brings into question the definition and the concept of deviance itself. Starting from the presupposition that the rules and their application do not constitute an objective and neutral reality, these theories do not have the goal of understanding why rules are violated, but aim instead to understand the processes by which deviance is defined, produced and used. In fact, the attempt to lead deviance in a deterministic way back to one or more previous causes has failed for various reasons; firstly because starting from the same initial conditions (neighborhood, family, lack of regulations) it is not necessary to develop a deviant behavior. Furthermore, the expectation of curing deviance like a disease includes the assumption that deviance itself could be separated from the rest of the society [46]. The traditional explanatory models, which identify antisocial and criminal behaviors with genetic and biological characteristics, with an inappropriate socialization and lacking internalization of the social rules, with personality disorders or with the social order (socioeconomic status, residence in degraded places, social and family disintegration, loss of values, etc.) are therefore left, in favor of interaction models [47]. Deviance is seen more as a path or a process than as the result or the effect of previous causes [48].

3.2.1. Symbolic Interaction

Symbolic interaction refuses the conception of reality that strictly separates deviant phenomena from normal phenomena, and criminals from non-criminals. Delinquency is considered as a broad behavior, not only among the individuals identified and punished by society. This perspective arises from G. H. Mead's [49] and Schutz's [50] thinking and highlights the symbolic character of human interactions, seeing deviance as a result of an interactive process between a subject who performs actions, regulations which establish the lawfulness of such actions, the social reaction to the infringement of rules and the modifications of the personal identity derived by the *labeling, stereotyping* and *exclusion* processes.

In the so-called neo-Chicagoans' works, Lemert [42], Becker [51], Erikson [52], Goffman [53] and Matza [54] replace the analysis of the causes with the examination of social and institutional processes of control and, in general, by the complex interaction between the deviant subject, rules and social reaction. From this perspective, human action takes on a sense related to symbolic meanings attributed by the individual. The “mind” and the “self” are no longer seen as innate elements, but as constructs defined by social context; through the communicative or symbolization process, individuals identify themselves and others. Symbols condition the way in which we see reality around us. From these concepts, there are the following ideas: for instance, a deviant act is intended in proceedings and dynamic terms; it can also be understood also in the light of social reaction, of the effects of penalty and of punitive measures on the perceiving of the self and of the stigmatizing character of some institutional procedures. As has been noticed, this perspective highlighted how deviance can be generated and how it develops, according to the interventions of institutions toward the deviant behavior, either pre-emptively or in terms of treatment [55].

Symbolic interaction drives the attention from the characteristics of the subject who commits a crime and from the social conditions that may lead to deviance, to the conflicting interaction between the request of the subject and the reaction of the living environment.

3.2.2. Labeling and Stigmatization Processes

To intervene in one of the components of the conflicts often means not to take into account how the conflict was provoked and, in many cases, especially not to take into account the effects on the individual. In many cases, the penalty, starting from social labeling and stigmatization processes, generates in the deviant subject a change in his public and private identity.

Stigmatization is "a process [that] leads to publicly mark people as morally inferior, through negative labels, stigmas [...] or public information" [56, 57]. Stigmatization makes the deviant share his stereotype as an essential and predominant of his own identity [58, 59]. Furthermore, being labeled as deviant has these consequences:

- a degradation of the *status*: the individual will be tagged as "delinquent", "mentally ill", "victim" and will be treated accordingly [60];
- the possibility of being recognized as a "*type*" of person;
- the acquisition of potentially transgressive and deviant knowledge, competences and abilities;
- the acquisition of a specific "mindset", with a following variation of hierarchy of values [56] and the possible affiliation to a "deviant subculture" [61, 62]. Isolation and self-marginalization, a characteristic of such groups, intensifies the deviant status of the belonging members;
- the non-necessity of representing himself in a normal and spontaneous way and the subsequent abandonment of other manifestations of the self. The deviant is induced to act in an unconventional way since there are no expectations for him to act normally;
- experimenting with the secondary benefits of his negative identity, either in terms of solidarity from other deviants or in terms of assistance and protection from some sectors of society. Giving to the deviant a permanent status and role gives them the right of being helped and assisted [62].

3.2.3. Deviance and Deviant Career: The Various Stages

The term "deviant career" was introduced in literature by Goffman [63] from his studies on the moral careers of mentally ill individuals, and was later extended by Becker [51] to deviant careers in general. Such conceptualization was later also applied to other forms of deviant careers, such as that of a gambler [64], drug abuser [65, 66], patients who suffer from psoriasis [67, 68], or patients who suffer from cancer [69].

This term describes a sequentially deviant model and prefigures a set of phases within the development of the deviant behavior; for each phase there is a change in the acts and in the perspectives of the individual. The concept of "career" is based on the idea of an intentional subject, who plays a main role in the origin and in the continuation of deviant activities.

The first step in the deviant's career consists in having access to a set of beliefs and ideas which can lead to the creation of transgressive situations, called also *historical-biographical antecedents* [12]. It is necessary that the subject, in specific circumstances, should be "willing" to put into action a specific behavior [51, 54], so that it is necessary for him to consider the deviant act as an opportunity. Regarding adolescents, the peer group is a "place of identification and communication" in which they exchange, define and invent ideas together, and which constitutes a sort of *cultural equipment* with which they face the sea of society out of the family environment [70, 71, 72].

When one of these acts takes place, breaking a rule or committing an abuse against others, it is important to understand the social reaction to that act. Within that reaction the processes of labeling and stigmatization, aforementioned, can be triggered and therefore can ascribe a meaning to that experience, triggering in the subject a self-reconsideration just in light of that meaning. This is the *phase of crisis*, in which the subject can discuss his own beliefs and identify new forms of self-representation. If, in conducting the reconsideration process, the subject develops strong motivations and deviant interests, he may turn deviance into his way of life, building his own identity around a transgressive life model.

We therefore witness a shift from a casual experience to a tested model (*consolidation phase*) of deviant activity, which is also defined through interaction with other deviant subjects [12]. In this phase, the individual raises his awareness of new types of experiences and starts to see them as meaningful for him. Therefore, the affiliation to a deviant group constitutes a real "conversion" of the individual [54], through which he reconsiders his own affinities and his cognitive and emotional constructs.

The implementation of such actions is therefore the result of a set of social experiences in which the individual learns those meanings, perceptions and judgments which make these activities desirable. Deviance is therefore a dynamic and productive process that goes through some phases in defining a real path to the deviant career.

4. Method Indications to Promoting Health

4.1. From Infringement as an Individual "Deviant" Act to the Conditions that Generated It (Co-Responsibility)

Another important feature of the question is the temptation of common sense to put insanity, mental illness and deviance together. In this case, as well, these are merely cultural beliefs that refer to constitutionalist theories, with a positivist imprint. These theories assume the existence of a causal relationship between psychopathological conditions and deviance. Psychopathological conditions can include either brain damage and cranial malformations, or psychological diseases. Even though there are still some who agree with such ideas, scientific studies have widely discredited this absolutist theory, asserting that the presence of a psychiatric diagnosis or of a psychological or existential disorder, even though it may be associated to a deviant act or violent behavior, does not constitute a decisive fact for those actions. Not every person affected by psychopathological, clinical disorders performs deviant or violent behaviors, just as individuals who perform deviant, or violent acts are not necessarily affected by psychological disorders. This is a common methodological mistake, which has also been made by scholars in the past; that is, dealing only with the "renowned" crime and not with the hidden one [7, 25, 51, 54]. In a school environment this issue takes on great value because, dealing only with the "crime" (for instance, insulting a teacher) means neglecting the conditions that made this crime possible within the class group. In many cases the choice of breaking the rules is not only made by an individual "affected" by psychological disorder; instead, the way in which people perceive the act of being together is related to how they perceive a certain institutional context and to how willing they are to break rules and pay the consequences of it. These are all elements of great relevance for engaging in a conversation with students, with the purpose of creating the possibility for them to make different choices or, as Rom Harrè says, different "narrative positioning". To intervene only regarding the deviant act means to neglect the cause that generated it, and the consequence of it merely involves looking for the culprit to punish him.

4.2. From Deviance as a Personal Feature to the Path of the Deviant Career

As we have seen, deviance is a complex and well-structured phenomenon that involves different dimensions, such as legal regulations. Depending on the regulations, violations may be different or may not occur. Therefore, if the will and the choices of the person who decides to deviate and the regulations of the surrounding context allow deviant acts, then attributing the complexity of such a phenomenon merely to deviant behavior is very reductive. Today scientific literature is more oriented toward examining how the "deviant career" – an expression similar to "professional career" – is carried out, referring to the journey in stages that leads the individual to the acquisition of illegal competences. Every stage is characterized by a specific psychological and social feature and entails a different approach within the surrounding context of the subject (school and other institutions). For every stage, there may be different intervention procedures, interventions of contrast and of deterrence, and there may be different operational strategies used. The path to implementation of the deviant career is, by definition, procedural and it may be hindered or facilitated according to the interactions with it. Scholars suggest that the deviant should not be considered in terms of his hypothetical personal characteristics but in terms of his goals and how much they contrast with the goals of the institution, so that the latter is encouraged to take action where it is needed the most [73]. Thus, intervention at school is both strategic and crucial because some deviant ideas can be hindered and some alternative careers can be supported.

4.3. From the Punishment of Deviant Behavior to Intentional Repair

Reflection on how to take action against transgressions or deviant acts is linked to the preceding arguments. In much international legislation, a difference exists between the justice mode for adults and for minors and to distinguish between their guidelines means to help schools in taking adequate action. Sanctions and rehabilitative systems are often part of the legislation for adults. The former aim to punish those who committed the crime or the transgression, especially by means of precautionary measures. This model is based on the principle, often constitutional, that the government ensures the punishment of the crime; in other words, "you do the crime, and you do the time". The belief of the legal administration is to consider the punishment as the best deterrent to crime. An example from the school context is a pupil's suspension for "insulting" a teacher. The second model, initially born as an integration of the first one, takes into account the rehabilitation of the individual; in other words, the subject has to be given the opportunity for social reinsertion, mainly through community work or through custody to social services. Such an approach is suggested by the idea that punishment is not enough for social reinsertion; rather, in respect to the latter, the punitive model is considered ineffective. In the school context, for instance, the class council decides to suspend the student who insulted the teacher and "sentences" him to carry out community work, which is helping the janitor to wash desks or classrooms. A critical aspect of this kind of approach is the lack of a close relationship between the transgression (crime) and the social rehabilitation (community work). In the latter example, what is the link between the act of cleaning the desks and the "insult to the teacher"? How can the action of helping the janitor develop in the perpetrator a more responsible attitude regarding teachers, school and community? The connection between the "infringement" and the punishment is purely a moral connection.

A different model from the two aforementioned is the restorative justice model [74, 75], which is based on researchers finding punishment to be ineffective and, rather, even intensifying the ideas of the deviant, just as prison or juvenile prison systematically treats the deviant. For example, many researchers assert that the symbolism associated with prison, both for what happens inside it and for the way in which someone is perceived when released, contributes to creating within the minor a self-representation increasingly exposed to deviance [76, 77, 78]. Such a model aims to create the conditions for the minor to make good the damage caused, from the commission of an infraction (or crime) to the assumption of responsibility for what he has done, whose main indicator is to implement actions opposing the infringement itself, thereby being socially and academically accepted. For instance, the idea of carrying out restorative actions can be shared with the student in respect to what has been committed for a designated period, ensuring that the student will not insult his teachers. The key tool is "probation", which implies a suspension of judgment, and punishment that will terminate in the event of repair and will be confirmed or increased in the event of recurrence.

REFERENCES

[1] Ladd, G. W., Kochenderfer, B. J., & Coleman, C. C. (1996). Friendship quality as a predictor of young children's early school adjustment. *Child Development,* 67, p. 1103–1118.

[2] Smink, J., & Schargel, F.P. (2004). *Helping Students Graduate: A Strategic Approach to Dropout Prevention. Larchmont*. New York: Eye on Education.

[3] Tilleczek, K. (2004). The illogic of youth driving culture. *The Journal of Youth Studies*, 7 (4), p. 479-493.

[4] Williams, K. D., Forgás, J. P. & von Hippel, W. (2005). *The Social Outcast: Ostracism, Social Exclusion, Rejection, & Bullying*. New York: Psychology Press.

[5] Estevez, E., Musitu, G., & Herrero, J. (2005). The influence of violent behavior and victimization at school on psychological distress: The role of parents and teachers. *Adolescence*, 40 (157), p.183-196.

[6] Chen, Y.F., In Wu, C., & Hsiu Lin, K. (2009). The dynamic relationships between parenting and adolescent delinquency: a group based model approach. *Crime and Criminal Justice International*, 12, p. 59-100.

[7] De Leo, G. (1998). *La devianza minorile. Il dibattito teorico, le ricerche, i nuovi modelli di trattamento*. Roma: Carocci.

[8] Bonino, S., Cattelino, E., & Ciairano, S. (2003). *Adolescenti e rischio.* Firenze: Giunti.

[9] Ezinga, M.A.J., Weerman, F.M., Westenberg, P.M., & Bijleveld, C.C.J.H. (2008). Early adolescence and delinquency: levels of personality development and self-control as an explanation of rule breaking and delinquent behaviour. *Psychology, Crime, and Law*, 14, (4), p. 339-356.

[10] Crosnoe, R., Erickson, K.G., & Dornbusch, S.M. (2002). Protective functions of family relationships and school factors on the deviant behavior of adolescent boys and girls-reducing the impact of risky friendships. *Youth Soc.* 33, p. 515–44.

[11] Millie, A. (2009). *Anti-Social Behaviour*. Maidenhead: McGraw Hill/Open University Press.

[12] von Cranach, M., & Harré, R. (1982). *The analysis of action. European Studies in Social Psychology*. Cambridge: Cambridge University Press.

[13] Bartol, C. R. (1999). *Criminal behavior: A psychosocial approach* (5th Ed.). Upper Saddle River, NJ: Prentice Hall.

[14] Okorodudu, G.N. (2010). Influence of parenting styles on adolescent delinquency in delta central senatorial district. *Edo Journal Of Counselling*, 3, (1), p. 58-86.
[15] Esmaeili, N.S., & Yaacob, S.N. (2011). Post-divorce parental conflict and adolescents' delinquency in divorced families. *Asian Culture and History*, 3 (2), p. 34-40.
[16] Can, G. (1990). *Factors affecting the self-concept of high school students*. Eskişehir: Anadolu Üniversitesi Basımevi.
[17] Harris-McKoy, D., & Cui, M. (2012). Parental control, adolescent delinquency, and young adult criminal behavior. *Journal of Child and Family Studies*, vol. 22 (6), p. 836-843.
[18] Bachman, J.G., Wadsworth, K.N., O'Malley, P.M., Johnston, L.D., & Schulenberg, J.E. (1997). *Smoking, drinking, and drug use in young adulthood: The impacts of new freedoms and responsibilities*. Mahwah, NJ: Lawrence Erlbaum.
[19] Demuth, S. & Brown, S.L. (2004). Family structure, family processes and adolescent delinquency: The significance of parental absence versus parental gender. *Journal Of Research in Crime And Delinquency*, 41, (1), p. 58-81.
[20] Siegel, A.W., & Scovill, L.C. (2000). Problem behavior: The double symptom of adolescence. *Development and Psychopathology,* 12, p. 763-793.
[21] Taylor, I., Walton, P., & Young, J. (1973). *The New Criminology: For a Social Theory of Deviance.* London: Routledge and Kegan Paul.
[22] Matza, D. (1964). *Delinquency and Drift*. New York: John Wiley.
[23] Lombroso, C. (1876). *L'uomo Delinquente* (The criminal man). Translated 1911 by Lombroso-Ferrero, G. Montclair, NJ: Patterson Smith.
[24] Garofalo, R. (1885). *Criminologia: studio sul delitto, sulle sue cause e sui mezzi di Repressione*. Torino: Bocca.
[25] De Leo, G., & Salvini, A. (1978), *Normalità E Devianza*. Milano: Mazzotta.
[26] Caplan, G. (1964). *Principles of Preventive Psychiatry*. New York: Basic Books.
[27] Segre S. (1997). *La devianza giovanile. Cause sociali e politiche di prevenzione*. Milano: F. Angeli.
[28] Contessa, G. (1994). *La prevenzione: teoria di modelli di psicosociologia e psicologia di comunità*. Milano: Cittàstudi edizioni.

[29] Peled, E. (1996). "Secondary" victims no more: Refocusing intervention with children. In J. L. Edleson & Z. C. Eisikovits (Eds.) *Future interventions with battered women and their families* (p. 125-153). Thousand Oaks, CA: Sage Publications.

[30] Tremblay, R.E., & Craig, W. (1995). Developmental crime prevention. In Tonry, M.& Farrington, D.P. (Eds.), *Building a safer society: Strategic approaches to crime prevention,* p. 151–236. Chicago: University of Chicago Press.

[31] Durkheim, E. (1933). *The Division of Labor in Society*. New York: Macmillan.

[32] Durkheim, E. (1951). *Suicide*. New York: Free Press.

[33] Parsons, T. (1937). *The Structure of Social Action: a study in social theory with special reference to a group of recent European writers*. New York: McGraw-Hill.

[34] Sutherland, E.H., & Cressey, D.R. (1960). *Principles of criminology*. Philadelphia: Lippincott

[35] Williams III, F.P., & McShane, M.D. (2004). *Criminological theory* (4th ed.). Upper Saddle River, NJ: Prentice Hall.

[36] Emler, N. & Reicher, S.D. (1995). *Adolescence and Delinquency*. Oxford: Blackwell.

[37] Merton, R.K. (1938). Social structure and anomie. In *American Sociological Review*, 3, p. 672−682.

[38] Merton, R.K. (1968). *Social Theory and Social Structure*. New York (NY): Free Press.

[39] Merton, R.K. (1973). *The Sociology of Science. Theoretical and empirical investigations*. Chicago: The University of Chicago Press.

[40] Cohen, A.K. (1955). *A general theory of subcultures. Delinquent boys: The culture of the gang*. New York: The Free Press.

[41] Cloword, R.A. & Ohlin Lloyd, E. (1960). *Delinquency and opportunity theory of delinquent gangs*. New York: The Free Pass.

[42] Lemert, E.M. (1951). *Social Pathology*. New York: Mcgraw-Hill.

[43] Bandura, A. (1973). *Aggression: a social learning analysis*. Englewood Cliffs (NJ): Prentice Hall.

[44] Bandura, A. (1977). *Social Learning Theory*. Englewood Cliffs (NJ): Prentice Hall.

[45] Bandura, A. (1986). *Social Foundations of Thought and Action*. Englewood Cliffs (NJ): Prentice Hall.

[46] Paternoster, R., & Brame, R. (1997). Multiple routes to delinquency? A test of developmental and general theories of crime. *Criminology*, 35, 49-84.
[47] De Wit, J., & van Der Veer, G. (1991). *Psychologie van de adolescentie. Ontwikkeling en hulpverlening*. Nijkerk: Uitgeverij.
[48] Berti C. (1997). La devianza adolescenziale, in Ravenna M. *Psicologia delle Tossicodipendenze,* Urbino: Il Mulino.
[49] Mead, G.H. (1934). *Mind, Self and Society.* Chicago: U of Chicago P.
[50] Schutz, A. (1962). Collected papers, 3 vols. *The Hague (Netherlands): Martinus Nijhoff.*
[51] Becker, H. S. (1963). *Outsiders*. New York: Free Pass.
[52] Erickson, M.H., & Rossi, E.L. (1982). *The Collected Papers of Milton H. Erickson of Hypnosis. Vol. I, II, III, IV: Hypnotic Investigation of Psychodynamic Processes*. New York: Irvington Publishers.
[53] Goffman, E. (1967). *Interaction Ritual*. Garden City, N.Y.: Anchor.
[54] Matza, D. (1969). *On Becoming Deviant*. Englewood Cliffs, NJ: Prentice Hall.
[55] Goffman, E. (1961) *Asylums: Essays on the Social Situation of Mental Patients and Other Inmates*. Garden City: Anchor Books.
[56] Lemert, E. (1967) *Human Deviance. Social Problems and Social Control.* Englewood Qiffs (New Jersey): Prentice Hall.
[57] Goode, E. (2004, March 9). Defying psychiatric wisdom, these skeptics say "prove it." *New York Times.*
[58] Salvini, A., (1998). *Psicologia Clinica*. Padova: Upsel Domeneghini Editore.
[59] Heatherton, T.F., Kleck, R.E., Hebl, M.R. & Hull, J.G. (2000). *The social psychology of stigma*. New York: Guilford Press.
[60] Moses, T. (2010). Adolescent mental health consumers' self-stigma: associations with parents' and adolescents' illness perceptions and parental stigma. *Journal of community psychology*, *38* (6), p. 781-798.
[61] Campbell, C., & Deacon, H. (2006). Unravelling the contexts of stigma: from internalisation to resistance to change. *Journal of community & applied social psychology*, 16 (6), p. 411-417.
[62] Link, B.G., & Phelan, J.C. (2001). Conceptualizing stigma. *Annual review of Sociology*, 363-385.
[63] Goffman, E. (1971): *Relations in Public: Microstudies of the Public Order*. New York: Basic Books.
[64] Hayano, D.M. (1982). *Poker Faces: The Life and Work of Professional Card Players*. Berkeley: University of California Press.

[65] Faupel, C. (1991) *Shooting Dope: Career Patterns of Hard-Core Heroin Users*. Gainesville: Univ. of Florida press.

[66] Dabney, D.A. & Hollinger, R.C. (2002). Drugged druggists: The convergence of two criminal career trajectories. *Justice Quarterly*, vol. 19, p. 201-233.

[67] Ginsburg, I.H., & Link, B.G. (1993). Psychosocial consequences of rejection and stigma feelings in psoriasis patients. *International Journal of Dermatology*, 32, p. 587-591.

[68] Ramsey, B., & O'Reagan, M. (1988). A survey of the social and psychological effects of psoriasis. *British Journal of Dermatology*, 118, p. 195-201.

[69] Bloom, J. R., & Kessler, L. (1994). Emotional support following cancer: A test of the stigma and social activity hypotheses. *Journal of Health and Social Behavior*, 35, p. 118-133.

[70] Altieri L., & Faccioli, P. (2002). Percezione delle norme sociali, trasgressione e devianza, in Buzzi C., Cavalli A., De Lillo A. *Giovani del nuovo secolo*. Bologna: il Mulino.

[71] Amerio, P., Boggi Cavallo, P., Palmonari A., & Pombeni, M.L. (1990). *Gruppi di adolescenti e processidi socializzazione*. Bologna: Il Mulino.

[72] Baraldi, C. (1988), *Comunicazione di gruppo. Una ricerca sui gruppi giovanili*. Milano: F. Angeli.

[73] Iudici, A., de Aloe S., Fornaro G., Priori, M., & Strada, A. (2014). Countering the "career of disability": from clinical institutionalization to the creation of opportunities for biographical change. The intervention of the Service for Integration, Accompaniment and Orientation for students with disabilities of the Municipalities of Melzo and Liscate (Mi). *Procedia- Social Behavioral Sciences*, Vol. 116, pag. 3271-3275. Elsevier Ltd.

[74] Braithwaite, J. (2002). *Restorative justice & responsive regulation*. Oxford: University Press.

[75] Van Ness, D. W., & Strong, K. H. (2013). *Restoring justice: An introduction to restorative justice*. Newnes.

[76] De Leo, G., & Patrizi, P. (2002). *Psicologia giuridica*. Bologna: Il Mulino.

[77] Iudici, A., Maiocchi, A. (2014). Community Justice and juvenile offender: the management of an individual case with criminal slope with community involvement. *Mediterranean Journal of Social Sciences*, Vol. 5 (20), pag. 2015-2027.

[78] Barbagli, M., & Gatti, U. (2005). *Prevenire la criminalità*. Bologna: Il Mulino.

Chapter 6

Bullying / Prevarication and School: Historical References, Concepts and Methods of Intervention

1. Introduction

Although the phenomenon that sees young people being repeatedly harassed by others is not new, bullying, as we know it, has been systematically studied only since the nineteen-seventies and mostly in some countries of northern Europe. Before properly addressing the subject of bullying, in psychology and sociology reference was made to aggression, and more specifically to forms of violent expression among peers.

It should be noted that, in researches and in scientific conceptualizations preceding the birth of the phenomenon, many scholars clearly refused the explanation of acts of violence among young people as expressions of innate elements which are therefore unchangeable. Aggressiveness among young people was configured more in social terms; for example, as the result of the apprehension of models and forms which were socially widespread, accepted and therefore reproducible in time [1, 2].

Lorenz [3] in the same period proposed a very articulated view of aggression, namely as the result of environmental factors and evolutionist factors. According to the author, without the "fighting instinct" the individual and the species could not ensure their own survival. Going back in time, we find an extremely utilitarian view of aggression. Merton [4, 5] suggested about twenty years earlier how it (and with it every other form of "deviance") represented an attempt of the disadvantaged social groups to obtain economic success and a social status that society unfairly reserved for other categories of people.

To confirm this view there are the techniques of neutralization and justification examined by Matza and Sykes [6], which would let the individual unload his own responsibility on that undefined body called community; such a process would justify violence among them.

However, what happened in Scandinavia in the early 1970s was a sort of proliferation of systematic studies to analyze the phenomenon in different terms; these studies initially gained interest especially in Sweden, a country where the public started to pay attention to these kinds of events just between the 1960s and '70s [7]. The attention started to head toward a more individualistic form of aggression, which shortly thereafter was named as bullying, enabling preventive interventions.

One of the events which, a little later, generated a peak of attention, as well as a series of chain reactions among the public and in institutions, took place in 1982, when it was announced through a newspaper that three Norwegian boys between ten and fourteen years of age had committed suicide after a series of acts of intimidation repeated over time by a group of peers.

This led, at the end of 1983, to the Norwegian Ministry of Education proposing a national campaign against this phenomenon in elementary and secondary schools in Norway [8]. The phenomenon is identified by the countries who first dealt with the argument in terms of *mobbing* (Norway and Denmark) or *mobbning* (Sweden and Finland). The original root of the English word "mob" refers to a group of people, usually large and anonymous, implicated in the actions of harassment. In the late eighties and early nineties, however, the phenomenon also affected other countries, including the UK, Canada, the USA, Japan and the Netherlands.

The term used by the Anglo-Saxons is bullying [9]. In any case, it should be noted that the value of the terms described suffers a great deal of the cultural contexts in which the phenomenon has been represented in different ways. The comparative study between countries is therefore hampered by the difficulties related to the translation of the term bullying, which in English means a well-defined behavioral phenomenology.

The major complications, despite the efforts of several authors, are because in countries like Spain, Portugal and Italy there are not any terms commonly used with a meaning equivalent to the English term [9, 10]. In Italy, scholars have translated the concept expressed by the Anglo-Saxon term with "prepotenza", trying to minimize the non-perfect equivalence of the two terms [11].

2. VIOLENT ACTS AT SCHOOL: RESEARCH CONTRIBUTIONS AND CLINICAL IMPLICATIONS

Some episodes of violence among peers in school which have emerged in the last twenty years have greatly increased the interest of the scientific community toward this phenomenon, which is then amplified and returned with tones of alarm to different social media. They have created new areas of research that have produced an extensive scientific literature that aims to identify the causes and characteristics, as well as methods of intervention to stem the flow, distributing responsibility among teachers, parents, society, media and personal characteristics.

At the international level, episodes of mistreatment, abuse and violence have been reported by several studies. In Spain and Norway, at least 15% of students in primary and secondary schools are involved in episodes of maltreatment among peers; in the UK it reaches 29% [12], Ireland 8%, and Canada 20% and in Israel not less than 60% of respondents [13]. In Italy, these episodes seem even more common among children than among adolescents [14, 15, 16, 17]. The fallout of such conduct may affect academic performance, interpersonal relationships, and self-representation and can generate anxiety or social phobia [18, 19, 20, 21, 22]. Violent behavior at school is also associated with various problems, such as being involved in brawls [23], youth suicide [24, 25], the consumption of alcohol or drugs [26, 27] and even psychopathological problems, such as eating disorders, depressive syndromes, and psychosomatic disorders [28, 29, 30], many of which are also treated pharmacologically [31]. In some studies an attempt to assess the long-term effect of aggressive behavior has been made [19, 20, 32]; however, the existence of real longitudinal studies is very limited. Also, the methodologies used to frame the variables are almost always based on questionnaires in which subjects are asked to respond for their own history, risking the collection of excessively personal reports on visions lacking objectivity, as long as we can speak of objective observations. Even regarding the collection of data on psychopathological conditions, there are unavoidable methodological problems; it happens that scales of behavior in which teachers and/or parents respond in place of those concerned are being used, providing subjective observations on the conduct of minors. This clearly makes the recognition of any symptoms hardly scientific, since the observations are provided by common sense.

Despite these data, the elements invoked to understand the aggressive actions between peers are various and depend fundamentally on the paradigmatic frames through which the phenomenon is being contextualized. While the school, the family and society as a whole are considered as key factors in the processes of socialization and then in the training and education of every young person, some studies have gone looking for personality characteristics that could reveal the existence of a deterministic phenomenon; others have given a specific weight to cultural elements through which one can understand the so-called process of peer prevarication, for which young people use aggressive manners. The first, causal-type, approach is still among the most popular, and within the latter were born many theories (and consequently intervention programs) to investigate certain elements that could explain the phenomenon. The second, the processual approach, is less common, both in terms of diffusion and in terms of the methodologies used; its purpose is to overcome some limitations of the first setting.

Aggressive actions among peers can therefore now be configured from two theoretical constructs, which outline two different ways of understanding the child:

1) The construct of bullying, formalized by the Swedish psychologist Dan Olweus [29, 33, 34, 35], which refers to the idea that aggression is, largely, genetically ingrained.
2) The construct of prevarication, which defines aggression among peers not in individualistic terms, but instead, as a product of a cultural process. Such a stance derives from the studies of other authors [36, 37, 38, 39, 40, 41, 42, 43, 44].

3. Bullying as Objective Fact: An Individualistic and Causal Approach to Aggressive Actions Among Peers

According to the famous definition of Olweus, considered the leading expert on the topic, bullying means "the offensive action of one or more arrogant individuals who act cruelly on weak individuals or on individuals with fewer resources in terms of physical strength and mental strength" [35]. The term "bullying" therefore outlines a situation in which "a student is the subject of bullying, i.e. he is being overcome or victimized, when exposed, repeatedly in the course of time, to the offensive actions implemented by one or more mates" [35].

In the definition of the scholar, we find that the phenomenon can be considered such in both cases when an individual harasses a fellow, and when a group of people implements actions. Another unique aspect is the fact that in this definition we are talking about students, as if to indicate that the phenomenon only affects the school environment; and actually we talk about bullying in literature in reference to school-age children (usually elementary and middle school) up to the stage of adolescence. The offensive acts in question may materialize through verbal abuse (such as insults, threats, persistent and unilateral teasing etc.), physical violence (such as beatings, public humiliation, aggression, domination by force, etc.) or indirect actions (such as exclusion from the group, refusing to fulfill requests, the disclosure of information which may be true or false, defamation, etc.) [11, 45, 46]. The asymmetry between the bully and the victim is a fundamental characteristic of bullying; students exposed to insults in fact should not be able to defend themselves, falling into a situation of powerlessness in the face of those who molest.

The literature differentiates between two forms of bullying: direct, which is characterized by overtly offensive actions against the victim, and indirect, which then consists of all those acts even more subtle and hidden that cause harm to the victim in a more complex way, for example, through the activation of negative reactions from others toward the victim [35].

In addition to the provided coordinates for guidance toward the individuation of episodes that make up what is called bullying, Olweus has focused much of his studies on determining the characteristics of bullies, in order to act on them in terms of prevention. The scholar defines bullies as children characterized by generalized aggression toward adults and peers, by impulsiveness and lack of empathy toward others in general. The behavior of a "bully" is referred to as a type of action (individual or collective), which aims to deliberately injure; it is often persistent, sometimes lasting for weeks, months and even years, and against which it is difficult for those who are victims to defend themselves. At the basis of most overpowering behaviors, there is an abuse of power and a desire to intimidate and dominate a peer, who can live in a condition of great suffering and marginalization [33]. The inclination of the bullies to commit violent behavior is provided on the one hand by the need for power and control, and on the other by a certain hostility toward the environment around them, often caused by inadequate family situations within which these subjects are raised [35]; this would explain the satisfaction that the bullies gain by inflicting suffering on others.

Many other authors have defined these individuals as having a general immaturity in recognizing emotions, especially positive ones [47]. Children who show bullying attitudes may be indicative of a general social maladjustment, which may subsequently lead to overt violence, or even crime [15].

Even regarding the victims, attempts have been made to identify those characteristics that seem to make up the profile type. Specifically, a description is provided of two types of victim, each with unique traits and tied to particular incidents of bullying: *passive* victims and *provocative* victims, of which the latter are rarer [45, 48, 49]. In the first type are included people who tend to be more anxious and insecure than the norm, individuals who present as quieter and more sensitive. These profiles are also characterized by low self-esteem and self-discrediting and devaluing visions. Another factor that seems to complete the picture is a certain lack of physical strength accompanied by negative attitudes toward violent acts; this would not explain bullying as being caused by provocations and/or harassing behavior of the victims. According to the author, the typical temperament and attitude of these subjects shows the inability of the latter to react to insults or attacks. This type of model is defined *reactive anxious or submissive*, associated (particularly for males) with physical weakness. Some in-depth interviews that the scholar has conducted with the parents of these students have shown that these youths have, since childhood, shown an overly prudent and cautious attitude, and heightened sensitivity [34]. Boys with these characteristics may have difficulty in affirming their status within the peer group, making them easy prey for various forms of aggression; this strengthens their already strong anxiety, insecurity and negative self-image [50]. Another element that emerges in Olweus' settings [49] is that these children during childhood have, compared to the average, a more intimate and positive relationship with their parents, which leads one to consider overprotection as both a cause and a consequence of bullying.

On the other hand, the provocative victims present themselves as subjects with a low concentration that leads them to behave in ways that irritate the majority of the class. These hyperactive subjects, which have a combination of both *anxious* and *aggressive* reactive models, cause the triggering of different dynamics compared to the case of the passive victims.

In summary, most of the features found in the scientific literature to define bullying, seen as offensive action, are:

1) First, importance is given to the relationship between peers. Bullying is closely associated with the youth culture of children; adults, therefore, are given the task of monitoring, preventing, combating or blocking acts of bullying by kids.
2) The second feature emerging from the studies in the literature is the disproportion of forces between aggressor and victim; bullying is different from a fight or clash between peers because the victim is helpless. In light of this reason, the consideration and the symbolic recognition of the «bully» are considered particularly relevant elements; the strongest or biggest, or the leader of the group, must prove their superiority to gain recognition within the group.
3) The third characteristic refers to the duration and continuity of the offensive act; bullying is not represented by an occasional act, but by a repeated and constant aggressive attitude.
4) Another aspect is whether the bully and the victim are identified by specific personal characteristics, which cause certain behaviors.

3.1. Interventions

The first interventions aimed at reducing bullying began in Scandinavia, when researchers began to look at the phenomenon more closely, implementing some serious consequences for harassment in schools [35], and derived from the settings exposed above. From the 1980s onwards, as already mentioned, there has been a growing interest in bullying in other countries, with the result that many researchers who began to attempt to respond to the alarm by developing the most diverse school programs [51, 52, 53, 54].

The institutions that deal with prevention feel the need to take action on bullying because this is considered a stable and especially objective phenomenon [51], which causes significant effects not only on the actors directly involved [18, 19, 20, 53], but also on peers who simply assist in it [56]. Starting from these motivations, what are the goals involved in the interventions in question, and to whom are they addressed? The main goals forming the basis of an intervention based on a paradigmatic causal matrix are the reduction of offending behavior among peers, the removal of the problems associated with it and the prevention of new episodes [57]. Such goals are usually pursued through a restructuring of the school environment [53, 58, 59, 60, 61, 62, 63]. In accordance with this arrangement, an informative approach is widely used, designed to divulge complete information on the phenomenon itself at all levels of the school education system [33].

Moreover, a greater disclosure of information allows teachers and parents to better recognize incidents of bullying. Many interventions are in fact based on increasing awareness about behaviors related bullying [24, 64, 65, 66, 67]. According to some authors, there is an understatement of the importance of bullying which, as an objective phenomenon, cannot be overlooked; at the same time there is an overestimation of the ability of victims to halt violence or face the episodes without the help of adults [53, 58]. Some programs have promoted policies of zero tolerance of bullying and have created spaces for counseling for offenders and victims [68, 69, 70].

3.2. Critical Aspects

As it is generally described and interpreted, this approach involves some critical aspects:

- First, the disproportionate relationship between forces seems to be a misleading and un-provable criterion, which leads to defining bullying through physical measurement of force rather than through the symbolic value of the bully, etc. In addition, the continuity of the offensive action that characterizes bullying, as defined above, has in fact no basis for standardization, while, in the attempt to evaluate this parameter, a theory would have the burden of establishing the standardized levels of continuity, removing them from the arbitrary assessment of victims or witnesses. Often the phenomena that come into the limelight as examples of bullying are specific episodes, of which you do not know the story, and for which it is therefore difficult to reconstruct the degree of repetition and frequency.
- The idea of a youth culture that produces offensive acts seems to be indefinite and uncertain. Studies on juvenile delinquency, particularly sociological ones, have long described gangs and the violent relationships within them, and acts of arrogance have been described in the interaction between the action of the leader, based on the recognition, and the support of the group. However, it is never referred to the individual, but through a social structure based on hierarchy, which is explicit and accepted as a predetermined regulatory framework, of which the offensive action is its direct

consequence [71, 72, 73]. In many situations identified as bullying, on closer inspection, the aggressive action does not seem to be generated by the effect of a hierarchical structure regulated and recognized by the participants; indeed, it seems to be the product of the ineffectiveness of the hierarchical structure, which, not being always accepted, must be continually set up. Many offensive actions become relevant when the bands do not have more success as a dominant cultural form [37].

- The marginal role assigned to adults (as we have said, the parents are involved to deter bullies, but in a few cases, it starts from their responsibility) is questionable, since it does not give an account of the importance of the social context in giving meaning to the offensive action. Configuring the offensive action as an unequal exchange between bully and victim means not considering the influence of the social context in concretely affecting the systems of collective communication; it seems that the rest of society has no direct contact with these groups of children and adolescents. The groups that are engaged in offensive actions and the rest of the group are treated as separate worlds, or rather, as related worlds in an obscure way. Given that communication is a circular process, it is quite clear that the forms of communication used by children and adolescents cannot be separated from those of adults [74].
- Even if standardized criteria were detected, a further difficulty would arise, as a theory of bullying based on statistical assumptions should ignore the comments of parents, teachers and victims, claiming, for example, that a random episode of offensive action is not bullying even if it is viewed as being particularly serious from the point of view of the social actors involved. In this regard, numerous studies highlight the diversity of perceptions between those of children living with bullying (acted or immediately) and scientific definitions. A major study seems to confirm that, in fact, the representation of "bullying" and "bully" typically seen in pre-adolescents corresponds only in part to the scientific representation of "bullying" [75]. In particular, among the features identified in literature as distinctive of "prevaricating behavior", the "recurrence" appears not to be associated with the "bully behavior" in almost half of the sample, and in the case of "asymmetry" of the bully-victim relationship, more than half of the sample does not consider it a defining factor of the "bully behavior". Swain [76], in this regard, spoke of "over-extension of the

definition of bullying", referring to how the subjects in childhood tend to associate numerous behaviors with "bullying", but not all are falsified.

4. The Culture of Prevarication: A New Paradigmatic Proposal

A different point of view, which differs from the viewpoint that bullying is attributable to the behavior and characteristics of a person, is defined by some scholars [36, 37, 40, 77, 78, 79, 80] who argue that the growing concern about this phenomenon is due to a culture of childhood that has become prevalent in today's society, consisting in modeling the behavior of children to adults, limiting and disregarding the deviations that may occur through a correctional approach.

From the ideas of these authors emerges the notion of how bullying embodies a concern of society rather than being an empirical object to be investigated, and constitutes the mirror of modern conceptions that do not recognize a child who assaults or who suffers. Therefore, if the available data describes events of this kind, it is necessary to observe them closely, monitor them and extrapolate the sickness concealed behind it, so that we can act in a preventive manner in an attempt to exorcise a reality perceived as dangerous, which turns into an enemy to be fought [36]. This attitude can lead to the child being considered as suffering from some "internal" disturbance, such as bullying.

Against this objective trend, Baraldi and Iervese [37] propose a reflection of a constructivist matrix, which casts doubt on the validity of a process that transforms a point of view into an "objective phenomenon".

The reasons that make it possible to doubt this objectivity are strongly correlated with each other. First and foremost is the same historicity of science, with its succession of paradigms, which reminds us that now we have begun to share the idea within the scientific community, there is no objectivity in facts, and there is no statute of reality, but there are a multitude of perspectives constructed by an observer. This concept initially made its way into modern physics, being called the Heisenberg uncertainty principle, and then passed into other disciplines, thanks to the reflections on Kuhn's Structure of Scientific Revolutions [81]. It is from these epistemological redefinitions that in the last three decades of the twentieth century a cognitive orientation has been established, according to which the facts of reality are interpreted as social constructs, which take form based on the consensus of many observers and of socially established verification systems [74, 82, 83, 84, 85]. The second reason is directly related to the first: those facts that are affirmed as objective, thanks to a consensus, are the result of a simplification, which seems to be formed in order to explain what becomes difficult to accept [37]. Here certainties become the result of these operations of simplification in response to an unsustainable doubt which is too difficult to entertain.

It is no coincidence that these are themes (such as bullying and ADHD) concerning childhood and adolescence, in whose interpretation the uncertainty of society appears to be particularly high and disturbing; the "fragility" and "weakness" of childhood and adolescence seem to put into question the future reproduction of society and of the human race [42, 86]. Society has in fact always tried to oppose the uncertainty generated by these two stages of life; pseudo-scientific speculations and interpretations are constructed in order to remove uneasiness generated by an unpredictability that calls into question the very future of society and of human beings.

The importance that currently affects the world of childhood and adolescence appears to be the result of some changes that have occurred in modern times in Europe [87]; in particular, the creation of a modern society differentiated by functions. From the social organizations of the Middle Ages (in hierarchical order) the evolution of layering evolved, structures with a specific role to meet specific needs were created, such as school, family, public services, justice, law enforcement, etc. [88]. It thus switched from the decisions taken by the King or the monarch to an organization based on systems and functions that help to regulate society.

According to this theoretical approach, childhood and adolescence have become particularly important because they represent those phases in which individuals acquire skills they can use in view of their future role in society. The purpose of socialization is to create a bridge between age categories and the organizational systems of adults. This is the case of a socialization that contemplates the acquisition in the current organizational system. This is, however, a specific socialization and does not seem to be the only one possible, but it is one of the possible paths of socialization.

From time immemorial, many of the most important scholars of childhood, such as Locke, Rousseau, Piaget, Vygotski, Freud and Bettelheim, have engaged in establishing psychosocial and developmental criteria aimed at trialing inclusion in society. Even sociology, psychology and pedagogy have been influenced by this explanatory trend, interpreting children primarily, if not exclusively, as a result of the causal mechanisms of socialization [89, 90]. The fact that the phenomenon in question worries scientists and researchers, teachers and parents, is related to the fact that the path of the child cannot be jeopardized by negative factors such as bullying; a child should be neither victim nor executioner. In simple terms, a child is not granted a deviant role from the principles and values imposed by society today, and if that happens, the deviance should be considered as an external body on which to act, a kind of virus to eradicate, to fight.

As a result of this social-cultural evolution, the anxieties and concerns for children and adolescents have also become particularly relevant; since childhood and adolescence are the stages in life at which one acquires functions and roles of responsibility, concern for the success of their acquisition becomes very high. Moreover, to justify such a failure, childhood and adolescence take on the characteristic of being periods of high vulnerability. Different types of socialization are explained by referring to the constructs of weakness and discomfort without questioning the current model of socialization [36].

Faced with the fear of failure within the proposed type of socialization, society activates forms of disengagement and self-appointed exemption, giving forms of deviance detached from itself the responsibility for the problems of children and adolescents [37]. From the point of view of the dominant, adult-centered culture, the child is not allowed to be either victim or aggressor; the certification of his innocence covers both sides. This implies that there is a great deal of attention paid to all of the phenomena which lead a child to become the victim or aggressor, which are regarded as external dangers to fight.

For this reason, bullying is presented as a phenomenon related to issues internal to groups of children; namely, there is the tendency to consider it a spontaneous or natural product of childhood. Nevertheless, this would be contrary to the studies themselves, firstly as this would be in flagrant contradiction with the dominant theories of development, according to which every aspect of relational life of the baby is connected to specific processes of socialization directed by the adult. Moreover, according to a constructivist perspective, violence, as an expression of communication, should be considered as a modality of offenses mediated by current cultural patterns. In this sense, the forms of offense are not disconnected from a specific sense socially and culturally ascribed. Children quickly learn to play and to fight by force; however, only when they learn the social rules of the offense do they become capable of using violence for purposes of coercion or oppression [43].

In other words, bullying requires some form of socialization to the social forms of injury and violence.

Several authors [37, 40, 41, 42, 44] have proposed thinking of bullying not as a phenomenon within the group of children, a natural element of childhood, but as a part of the general array of possible and, of course, contestable social roles. Specifically, implementation of violent and arrogant behavior can be seen, according to this viewpoint, as the result of a social construction of the child as an adult: "the violent child becomes adult because on the latter is projected a *culture of offense* born in the existing company" [37]. Alanen [91] states that "generationing" refers to the process through which one individual is construed as being a "child" and the other individual as an "adult", which has major consequences for the activities and identities of the members of each of those categories, but also their mutual relationships.

Scientific interest should therefore address not so much the offensive action in itself, but those cultural processes that prepare, accompany and legitimize, making it ongoing. The authors who propose this approach suggest the use of the term *prevarication* to refer to what originates the offensive action and what makes it reproducible; in fact, the prevarication can include it, but cannot run out in it. As already mentioned, another critical aspect of the classic conceptualizations of bullying is the fact that often this phenomenon is attributed to the specific context of childhood and the relationships between peers, as if the world of adults, and society as a whole, had nothing to do with the issue in question. This view contrasts with the argument that the forms of communication between children and adolescents are closely related to those between youths and adults, which is why one cannot think about the outside world, childhood and adolescence as neutral factors that do not come into play in the implementation of offensive and violent actions.

The introduction of these conceptual categories allows us to observe that:

1) Rather than an offensive action, prevarication is characterized as a symbolic system of allocation of deviant roles and attributions of meaning to actions;
2) Rather than a product of the culture of children, prevarication is characterized as the product of the combination of the culture of children and the culture produced in communication with adults;
3) Rather than by the disproportion of forces, prevarication is facilitated by the lack of legitimacy of hierarchical rules;

4) Instead of the continuity of the offensive action, prevarication is characterized by the importance assigned to offensive action by the participants;
5) Rather than as a causal factor, prevarication is characterized as the cultural field generator of ideas, narratives and definitions of reality capable of introducing and justifying offensive actions [42].

In this sense, prevarication is not observed only or mainly in the forms of communication that precede violent action, but also and especially in those that follow, making its reproduction likely; that is, the reactions to the offensive action [92]. The goal is to understand the success of the offensive action, not its manifestation; prevarication is not primarily important as a cause of offensive action, but rather as a cultural form, which makes its reproduction likely. On the other hand, looking for the cause - assuming that it is epistemologically correct - does not increase the chance that you can avoid the phenomenon of violent or aggressive acts, as the relationship between cause and effect is not reflected in the actions and intentions [93].

Summing up, then, the object of this proposal is outlined as a cultural form that guides and influences the communication, which produces the negation of the person affected by offensive acts and involves not only the protagonists of the act but also all those who witness it through the reactions to that event.

5. Method Indications To Promoting Health

To understand prevarication as a cultural process means to analyze the ways in which children, adolescents and adults trigger offensive actions. Consequently, in this setting new conceptual categories become central. The fundamental cultural components on which understanding of the processes of prevarication is based are: the manner of the offensive action; the social roles assigned to the adults in the construction of the prevarication; and the role of the educational system.

5.1. Since the Action Because the Offensive as It Occurs

Too often, researches that have dealt with bullying have attempted to identify the causal mechanisms underlying the bullying, especially trying to investigate the personality characteristics of victims and aggressors. Consequently, using the same approach, the focus has shifted to the long-term effects of bullying, trying to broaden the knowledge on what appears to be a concatenation of causes and consequences.

Various explanations of the offensive behavior of children call into question mainly the characteristics of the aggressor and/or victim (cognitive deficits, excessive insecurity, hyperactivity, etc.). The school environment (poor control of some places, school personnel either absent or not competent etc.), or the relationships between peers (oriented to injure, established by hierarchies, promoted from bad influences, etc.).

Through an epistemological reflection involving health promotion, it emerges that offensive or arrogant actions do not have an empirical-factual equivalent and do not refer to mechanical properties. Therefore, the causal view seems not to be relevant in the face of the sphere of social sciences, in which the meanings attributed and the symbolic specificity inherent in the language constitute an even more complex event which is not reducible to objective causes [94].

In view of this, a change of course is necessary to shift the focus from an attempt to provide an explanation of the phenomenon of "bullying" to an approach oriented toward understanding how the specific components of the detected situation (students, classes, teachers, parents) contribute in the generation of the situation itself, and especially how they share the management of joint responsibility for it.

After all, the intervention on the prevarication is independent of the reported case or the seriousness of it; it is interested in either identifying perpetrators or stigmatizing behaviors. Given that adolescents implement behaviors which derive from the ideas, concepts and theories in the context of cultural belonging, we can express an analogy in which the so-called bully is to the aggressive action as the actor is to the context of acting.

5.2. From Childhood as an Inherent Problem to the Co-Responsibility between Different Roles

In studies concerning the traditional "bullying", as we have seen, the intervention is carried out mainly on the universe of childhood and/or adolescence, taking into account the role of adults solely with respect to any responsibility for supervision, control and surveillance in environments where it is more common for events related to the phenomenon to occur. They are assigned the primary or exclusive role of acting or reacting against bullying; as a result, we try to provide them with tools for intervention, both preventive and correctional [42]. Hence, the continual proliferation of brochures and manuals that prescribe helpful tips for parents and teachers. Nevertheless, these tools can be effective if you have not previously understood how the participation of adults in communication with children and adolescents has or has not contributed to the culture of prevarication.

Rarely do we read that the influence of the adult world has contributed to the occurrence of bullying, in particular, the influence of the parents and teachers, and the methods they use to hinder the episodes [95]. It seems that people want to "shift" the entire blame onto the world of children, segregating it and isolating it to prevent the adults from feeling guilty of a fault. If one adopts an interaction and constructivist perspective, however, one cannot help but involve the complexity of the environment, observing every negotiation that would give meaning to an action for prevarication, and retracing it. Through this framework communication styles between parents and with children also become relevant, just as the way in which a teacher handles his or her role and interacts with the class also becomes important; in fact, it appears untenable and contrary to all theories of development to shift the whole blame onto children and their characteristics, as if their universe was isolated from that of adults and independent from the negotiation of meanings, including those that enable offensive acts.

From this point, the change in perspective lies in the refocusing of attention from childhood/adolescence, understood as an inherent problem, to the responsibilities of all actors involved. Consequently, the child is only one part in the game, and the adults share the responsibility for having contributed to the generation of offensive actions. In this logic, it is not possible to identify a cause, nor a culprit, nor even to consider that the problem is only one part, being childhood or adolescence. It is about giving up reductionist logic, as has been described above, and also building an intervention project shared between all the parties, aimed at generating changes in all the actors.

5.3. The Empowerment of Parents

If actions against "bullying" are organized in such a way as to prevent the offensive action or behavior of the "bully", in the approach of the "culture of prevarication", there is no reason for prevention to exist, as the culture, like a cold, cannot be avoided. Therefore, what matters is to understand what procedures the people involved (and institutions) use in promoting, directly or indirectly, or in contrasting situations of prevarication. As for the parents, it is necessary to identify the correct stance to take when facing this type of situation, either in specific cases or hypothetical ones. What are the prevailing theories? Should one justify the episodes? Should one justify the prevarication as a means of defence, or only in terms of reaction? Should one understate the offense, or blame the teachers, or the Headmaster? They are able to share a project with other roles? Should they blame the behavior solely on the children, and then use authoritarian methods of discipline against them? These are just a few questions designed to develop understanding of the contribution that parents make to the culture of prevarication, both in the generation of specific situations, and in terms of the design of an intervention shared with other actors.

5.4. The Responsibility of the School

Again, from the perspective of a culture of prevarication, it is necessary to investigate which modality uses the educational institution to deal with situations of prevarication, both in terms of organization and the way in which teachers and leaders exercise their roles. The relationships between the members of the school (students, teachers, parents) have historically been set based on educational criteria, identified almost exclusively in the process of education. The regulative principles of the educational process are summarized as follows: 1) the relationship between teachers and students is asymmetrical, both in terms of knowledge and in terms of the role; 2) assessment is one-sided (always through the formulation of questions, tasks and exams) and is based substantially on the metric system; 3) there is no customization of teaching, except for persons certified as having special educational needs. Therefore, students are regarded as being equal to one another. The educational organization is defined in classes and students are forced to stay together. Often there is a strong moral pressure from adults for students to "get along and be united" and if this does not occur, they attribute judgments, such as it being a bad class or a noisy class, etc. Furthermore, there is no duty to provide training for teachers on the management of groups, for example, a competence in which the majority of teachers have never followed any course.

It is important to point out that this approach was born in a different historical period, in which there were other needs of society, families, students, and citizens. The relational patterns that result from the aforementioned process of education were not only recognized, but also desired and appreciated by the entire community. Today, the same scheme is discussed and disputed by many, from which arguments there follows a de-legitimization of the entire institution of the school.

As you can see, the dynamics created by that organization, in fact, produce some problems: 1) First, in this context, a child or a preteen who feels uncomfortable or out of place in the class has little chance to 'get out', as he could in a system of voluntary attendance, and must necessarily suffer all the consequences, among which there is also the possibility of becoming a victim or aggressor; 2) secondly, the asymmetry of roles, if not anchored to specific objectives, risks configuration in terms of power and insubordination of the student to the educational intentions of teachers. It is often believed that children in classrooms, and particularly pre-adolescents, should be calm and learn in silence; they have to perform a role in which their opinion is irrelevant. On closer inspection, these conditions expose much to a culture of prevarication, because the interactive and relational dynamics are based neither on comparison, nor on sharing. Formal education establishes an implicit denial of all aspects of the children which are not related to the dynamics highlighted above, and in some cases rejects the affective, relational, social and cultural life of the classroom, creating even among peers a primary orientation to role relations of a regulatory model. A concrete example is the almost absolute use of surnames to identify individuals in secondary schools.

This particular instructional format is followed by a socialization of pupils to being disinterested in exploring other aspects of their peers, thus creating favorable conditions for the culture of prevarication. The school system can in fact generate the conditions for a deviation from its internal function, not through a fault, but through the routine, which is its daily organization. We must therefore admit that often offensive acts may become a form of deviance integrated into and produced from the educational processes involved in the school context. It is therefore no coincidence that the culture of prevarication asserts itself primarily in the education system. The deviant integration is a "physiological" consequence of a depersonalized form of education based on cognitive-normative criteria, which may not differentiate between outside, the "park", or the playroom.

Referring to the role of teachers, it is necessary to analyze how they orient themselves in situations of prevarication. What do they think? How do they act? What methods do they consider useful to hinder the offensive action? The punitive sanctionary model? The restorative model? The moralistic one? The correctional one? Are they blaming it entirely on the family? Or on their colleagues? On society, which they see as distinct from the school? Do they take responsibility for identifying appropriate strategies? Are they able to do so in-group (including teachers) and compared to the group (class)? Are they able to detect their own errors? Does the school organization allow them to work on this themselves? Do they feel that they have to deal only with curricular subjects?

5.5. From the Attribution of the Label of "Bully" to the Attribution of Roles Shared with the School Institution

As we have already argued, offensive acts are only one non-relevant aspect to the understanding of the whole phenomenon, because they represent only the tip of a problem. The offensive action cannot therefore be attributed causally to peers or to the individual because the prevarication is not a cultural form belonging to a single group, but is produced in the interaction between children, adults and the social-cultural environment. From our perspective the offensive action, and especially how it is "narrated" by those involved, is nothing less than the best possible solution that the child decided to implement in that given context, particularly from the point of view of expression (what the gesture or action means to communicate or communicates) and instrumental (the effects on who performs the action, the symbolic benefits that the action contains). Its implementation is also in relation to the possibilities conferred by the same context: others agreed with my action; the institutional reactions are worth less than my interests; the symbolic value of the action matters more than a thousand disciplinary notes, etc. In this case, the theatrical analogy is relevant; therefore, the prevaricator is to the offensive action as the actor is to his script (not meaning the script in individualistic terms).

In accordance with this, the specificity of an intervention in the school context should therefore apply to all pupils in the class (and in many cases the school) and not directly to the "bullies" and their "victims", in order to favor a stable and permanent change derived from a different relational choice. Moreover, as has been stated several times now, the identification of the "bully" shall be assigned to a static and stigmatized role, with the effect of inducing a self-representation based exclusively on the role that you actually want to hinder, and a collective vision focused on the aggressor only as a "bully". The consequence is that the subject identifies himself fully in that role, stigmatizing his actions even more, and setting more and more down the relational process between himself and others.

From our perspective, we should focus all efforts on how to induce a change in perspective in relation to the acts of prevarication. This means "to peel" the presence of static roles, such as "bully" or "victim." If this is the goal, then it may be useful first to detect the narrative position of the subject; for example, to understand which ideas allow that specific structuring of roles in which he or another prevails. It is useful to identify which naive theory the child uses to relate to the act of prevarication. Does he justify his action? What reasons are given when he decides to prevaricate? On which ideas is the abuse act founded? What does he want to achieve through that action? What can hinder these ideas? What can instigate them, both in the intervention of the family and in that of the teachers and his companions? How can pupils be involved in the analysis of the critical situation? How can the management of this situation be shared with them? What skills are active in the context of the class and which can be developed? What role is more useful to involve in intervening with prevaricators and with the whole class? The ultimate goal is to induce the shift from the role of "bully" to that of one who participates, analyzes, shares, and changes; that is, to take instead one of the roles that is allowed and desired by the school and the community.

References

[1] Bandura, A., Ross, D., & Ross, S.A. (1961). Transmission of aggression through the imitation of aggressive models. In *Journal of Abnormal and Social Psychology*, 63 (3), p. 575-582).

[2] Bandura, A., Ross, D., & Ross, S.A. (1963). Imitation of film-mediated aggressive models. In *Journal of Abnormal and Social Psychology*, 66 (1), p. 3-11.

[3] Lorenz, K. (1963). *On Aggression*. San Diego (CA): Harcourt Brace.

[4] Merton, R.K. (1938). Social structure and anomie. In *American Sociological Review*, 3, p. 672–682.

[5] Merton, R.K. (1973). *The Sociology of Science. Theoretical and empirical investigations*. Chicago: The University of Chicago Press.

[6] Matza, D., & Sykes, G.M. (1957). Techniques of Neutralization: a Theory of Delinquency. In *American Sociological Review*, 22 (6), p. 664-670.

[7] Heinemann, P.P. (1972). *Mobbning-gruppvald bland darn och vuxna.* Stockholm: Natur och Cultu.

[8] Pepler, D., & Rubin, K. (2013). *The development and treatment of childhood aggression.* Hillsdale (NJ): Erlbraum.

[9] Menesini, E., & Giannetti, E. (1997). *Il questionario sulle prepotenze per la popolazione italiana: problemi teorici e metodologici.* Firenze: Giunti.

[10] Smith, D. (1992). The incidence and nature of cross-sex bullying amongst pupils of junior school age. In *Education today*, 42 (2), p. 31-36.

[11] Genta, M.L., Menesini, E., Fonzi, A., Costabile, A., & Smith, P.K. (1996). Bullies and victims in schools in central and southern Italy. *European Journal of Psychology of Education*, 11(1), 97-110.

[12] Nansel, T.R., Overpeck, M., Pillla, R., Ruan, W.J., Simons-Morton, B., & Schedt, P. (2001). Bullying behaviours among US youth: prevalence and association with psychosocial adjustment. In *The Journal of American Medical Association,* 25, 285 (16), p. 2094-2100.

[13] Gofin, R., Palti, H., & Mandel, M. (2002). Fighting among Jerusalem adolescents: personal and school-related factors. In *Journal of Adolescent Health*, 27 (3), p. 218-223.

[14] Fonzi A. (a cura di) (1996). Disagio giovanile a scuola: programmi di ricerca e intervento. In *Età evolutiva*, 53, p.7 0-89.

[15] Fonzi, A. (1997). *Il bullismo in Italia*. Firenze: Giunti.

[16] Menesini, E. (2000). *Bullismo. Che fare?* Torino: Giunti.

[17] Menesini, E. (a cura di) (2003). *Bullismo: le azioni efficaci della scuola.* Trento: Erikson.

[18] Leymann, H. (1990). Mobbing and psychological terror at workplaces. In *Violence and Victims*, 5, p. 119-126.

[19] Smith, P.K. (1997). Bullying in life-span perspective: what can studies of school bullying and workplace bullying learn from each other? In *Journal of Community and Applied Social Psychology*, 7, p. 249-255.

[20] Lyznicki, J.M., McCaffree, M.A., & Robinowitz, C.B. (2004). Childhood Bullying: Implications for physicians. In *American Family Physician*, 70, p. 1723-1730.

[21] Rivers, I. (2004). Recollections of bullying at school and their long-term implications for lesbians, gay men and bisexuals. In *Crisis,* 24, p. 169-175.

[22] Tehrani, N. (2004). Bullying: A source of chronic posttraumatic stress? In *British Journal of Guidance and Counselling*, 32, p. 357-366.

[23] Kim, Y.S., Leventhal, B., Koh, Y., Hubbard, A., & Boyce, T. (2006). School bullying and youth violence. Causes or consequences of psychopathologic behavior? In *Archives of General Psychiatry*, 63, p. 1035-1041.

[24] Unnever, J.D. (2005). Bullies, aggressive victims, and victims: are they distinct groups? In *Aggressive Behavior*, 31, p. 153-171.

[25] Brunstein Klomek, A., Marrocco, F., Kleinman, M., Schonfeld, I.S., & Gould, M.S. (2007). Bullying, depression and suicidality in adolescents. In *Journal of the American Academy of Child and Adolescent Psychiatry*, 46, 1, p. 40-49.

[26] Loeber, R., & Dishion, T. (1983). Early predictors of male delinquency: a review. *Psychological bulletin*, 94 (1), 68.

[27] Magnusson, D., & Bergman, L.R. (1988). Individual and variable-based approaches to longitudinal research in early risk factors. In M. Rutter (Ed.), *Studies of psychosocial risk: The power of longitudinal data* (pp. 45–61). New York: Cambridge University Press.

[28] Parker, J.G., & Asher, S.R. (1987). Peer relations and later personal adjustment: are low accepted children at risk? In *Psychological bulletin*, 102, p. 457-489.

[29] Olweus, D. (1994). Annotation: bullying at schools: basic facts and effects of a school based intervention program. In *Journal of Child Psychology and Psychiatry*, 35, p. 1171-1190.

[30] Rivers, I., & Smith P.K. (1993). Types of bulling behaviour and their correlates. In *Aggressive Behaviour*, 20, p. 259-368.

[31] Sourander, A., Ronning, J., Brunstein-Klomek, A., Gyllenberg, D., Kumpulainen, K., Niemelä, S., Helenius, H., Sillanmäki, L., Ristkari, T., Tamminen, T., Moilanen, I., Piha, J., & Almqvist, F. (2009). Childhood bullying behavior and later psychiatric hospital and psychopharmacologic treatment. Findings from the Finnish 1981 birth cohort study. In *Archives of General Psychiatry*, 66, 9, p. 1005-1012.

[32] Einarsen, S., & Raknes, B.I. (1997). Harassment in the workplace and the victimization of men. In *Violence and Victims*, 12, p. 247-263.

[33] Olweus, D. (1991). Bully/victim problems among schoolchildren: basic facts and effects of a school based intervention program. In Pepler, D., Rubin, K., *The development and treatment of childhood aggression.* Hillsdale (NJ): Erlbraum.

[34] Olweus, D. (1993). *Bullying at school. What we know and what we can do*. Oxford: Blackwell Publishers.

[35] Olweus, D. (1993). *Bullying at school. What we know and what we can do.* Oxford: Blackwell Publisher. (trad. it *Bullismo a scuola*. Firenze: Giunti, 1996, p. 11)

[36] James, A., Jenks, C., & Prout, A., (1998). *Theorising childhood. Cambridge*: *Polity,*

[37] Baraldi, C., & Iervese, V. (2003). *Come nasce la prevaricazione. Una ricerca nella scuola dell'obbligo.* Roma: Donzelli Editore.

[38] Corsaro, W.A. (1997). *The sociology of childhood. Thousand Oaks*: Pine forge press.

[39] Chisholm, L., Buchner, P., Kroger, H.H., & Bois-Reymond, M. du (Eds.) (1995). *Growing up in Europe. Contemporary Horizonsin Childhood and Youth Studies*. Berlin/New York: Walter de Gruyter.

[40] Baraldi, C., & Rossi, E. (2002). *La prevenzione delle azioni giovanili a rischio*. Milano: F. Angeli.

[41] James, A., & Prout, A. (1997). *Constructing and reconstructing childhood: Contemporary issues in the sociological study of childhood.* London: Routledge.

[42] Iudici, A., De Aloe, S. (2006). Dal bullismo alla prevaricazione: un cambiamento paradigmatico in *Il volto nascosto della Delinquenza*. (A cura di) Pisapia, G.V. (p. 113-134). Torino: UTET Edizioni

[43] [43] Iudici, A., de Aloe, S. (2009). Bullismo o prevaricazione? Un cambiamento paradigmatico. In Confalonieri E., Cannone S., Martelli C. (A cura di), *Psicologia e Scuola* (p. 206-214). Trento: Erickson.

[44] Jenks, C. (1996). *Childhood*. London: Routledge.

[45] Björkqvist, K., Ekman, K., & Lagerspetz, K. (1982). Bullies and victims: their ego picture, ideal ego picture and normative ego picture. In *Scandinavian Journal of Psychology*, 23 (1), p. 307-313.

[46] Rivers, I. (2004). Recollections of bullying at school and their long-term implications for lesbians, gay men and bisexuals. In *Crisis*, 24, p. 169-175.

[47] Veltkamp, L. J., & Lawson, A. (2008). Impact of Trauma in School Violence on the Victim and the Perpetrator: A Mental Health Perspective. In *School Violence and Primary Prevention*, pp. 185-200.

[48] Olweus, D. (1973). *Hackkycklingar och översittare. Forskining om skol mobbning*. Stockholm: Almqvist & Wicksell.

[49] Olweus, D. (1978). Aggressions in the schools. In *Aggressive Behaviour*, 5 (3), p. 309-311.

[50] Schwartz, D., Dodge, K.A., Pettit, G.S., & Bates, J.E. (1997). The early socialization of aggressive victims of bullying. In *Child Development*, 68, p. 665–675.

[51] Pepler, D., Craig, W., Ziegler, S., & Charach, A. (1994). A school-based anti-bullying intervention: preliminary evaluation. In *Canadian Journal of Community Mental Health*, 13 (2), p. 95-110.

[52] Salmivalli, C., Kaukiainen, A., & Voeten, M. (2005). Anti-bullying intervention: Implementation and outcome. *British Journal of Educational Psychology*, 75 (3), p. 465-487.

[53] Olwues, D., & Limber, S.P. (2010). Bullying in school: evaluation and dissemination of the Olweus Bullying Prevention Program. In *American Journal of Orthopsychiatry*, 10 (1), p. 124-134.

[54] Battey, G.J.L. & Ebbeck, V. (2013). A qualitative exploration of an experiential education bully prevention Curriculum. *Journal of Experiential Education*, 36 (3), p. 203-217.

[55] Ayenibiowo, K.O., & Akinbode, G.A. (2011). Psychopathology of bullying and emotional abuse among school children. In *Ife Psychologia*, 19 (2), p. 127-141.

[56] Cummings, E., Vogel, D., Cummings, J.S., & El-Sheikh, M. (1989). Children's responses to different forms of expression of anger between adults. In *Child Development*, 60 (6), p. 1392-1404.

[57] Olweus, D., Limber, S.P., Flerx, V., Mullin, N., Riese, J., & Snyder, M. (2007). *Olweus Bullying Prevention Program: schoolwide guide*. Center City (MN): Hazelden.

[58] Pepler, D.J., Craig, W.M., & Roberts, W.L. (1998). Observations of aggressive and nonaggressive children on the school playground. *Merrill-Palmer Quarterly*, 44, 55-76.

[59] Melton, G.B., Limber, S.P., Cunningham, P., Osgood, D.W., Chambers, J., Flerx, V., & Nation, M (1998). *Violence among rural youth. Final report*. Washington (DC): U.S. Department of Justice, Office of Justice Programs, Office of Juvenile Justice and Delinquency Prevention.

[60] Bauer, N., Lozano, P., & Rivara, F.P. (2007). The effectiveness of the Olweus Bullying Prevention Program in public middle schools: a controlled trial. In *Journal of Adolescent Health*, 40, p. 266-274.

[61] Black, S.A., & Jackson, E. (2007). Using bullying incident density to evaluate the Olweus Bullying Prevention Programme. In *School Psychology International*, 28, p. 623-638.

[62] Pagliocca, P.M., Limber, S.P., & Hashima, P. (2007). *Evaluation report for the Chula Vista Olweus Bullying Prevention Program.* Final report prepared for the Chula Vista, CA, Police Department.
[63] Glew, G.M., Fan, M.Y., Katon, W., & Rivara, F.P. (2008). Bullying and school safety. *The Journal of pediatrics*, 152 (1), p. 123-128.
[64] Holt, M.K., & Espelage, D.L. (2007). Perceived social support among bullies, victims, and bully-victims. In *Journal of Youth Development*, 36, p. 984-994.
[65] Leff, S.S. (2007). Bullying and peer victimization at school: considerations and future directions. In *School Psychology Review*, 36, p. 406-412.
[66] Reid, P., Monsen, J., & Rivers, I. (2004). Psychology's contribution to understanding and man-aging bullying within schools. In *Educational Psychology in Practice*, 20, p. 241-258.
[67] Smith, P.K. (2004). Bullying: recent developments. In *Child and Adolescent Mental Health*, 9, p. 98-103.
[68] Hunt, C. (2007). The effect of an education program on attitudes and beliefs about bullying and bullying behavior in junior secondary school students. In *Child and Adolescent Mental Health*, 12, p. 21-26.
[69] Smokowski, P.R., & Kopasz, K.H. (2005). Bullying in school: an overview of types, effects, family characteristics, and intervention strategies. In *Children & Schools*, 27, p. 101-110.
[70] Souter, A., & McKenzie, A. (2000). The use and effects of anti-bullying and anti-harassment policies in Australian schools. In *School Psychology International*, 21, p. 96-105.
[71] Pitch, T. (1982) *La devianza*. Firenze: la Nuova Italia.
[72] De Leo, G., & Salvini, A. (1978). *Normalità e Devianza*. Milano: Mazzotta.
[73] De Leo, G. (1990). *La devianza minorile*. Roma: Nis.
[74] Watzlawick, P. (1984). *The invented reality: Contributions to constructivism*. New York: W.W. Norton.
[75] Caravita, S., & Ardino, V. (1998). Rappresentazione del comportamento prepotente e del "prepotente". *Archivio di Psicologia Neurologia e Psichiatria*, 59 (5), p. 554-566.
[76] Swain, J. (1998). What does bullying really mean? *Educational Research*, 40, 3, p. 358-364.
[77] Woodhead, M. (1997). Psychology and the cultural construction of children's needs. In James, A., & Prout, A. (Eds.). *Constructing and*

reconstructing childhood: Contemporary issues in the sociological study of childhood, p. 63-84.

[78] Hallett, C., & Prout, A. (Eds.). (2003). *Hearing the voices of children: Social policy for a new century*. London: Routledge.

[79] Alderson, P., & Morrow, V. (2004). *Ethics, social research and consulting with children and young people*. Barkingside: Barnardos.

[80] James, A., & James, A. (2004). *Constructing childhood: Theory, policy and social practice*. Basingstoke: Palgrave Macmillan.

[81] Kuhn, T. (1969). *La struttura delle rivoluzioni scientifiche*. Torino: Einaudi.

[82] Salvini, A., (1998). *Psicologia Clinica*. Padova: UPSEL Domeneghini Editore.

[83] Maturana, H. & Varela, F. (1986). *The tree of knowledge: the biological roots of human understanding*. Boston, MA: New Science Library.

[84] Bateson, G. (1972). *Steps to an ecology of mind: Collected essays in anthropology, psychiatry, evolution, and epistemology*. University of Chicago Press.

[85] Ceruti, M., & Bocchi, G. (1985). *La sfida della complessità*. Milano: Feltrinelli.

[86] Iudici, A., Faccio, E., Belloni, E. Costa, N. (2014). The Use of the ADHD Diagnostic Label: What Implications Exist for Children and Their Families? In *Procedia- Social Behavioral Sciences*, vol. 122, p. 506-509.

[87] Aries, P. (1968). *Padri e figli nell'Europa medievale e moderna*. Bari: Laterza.

[88] Luhmann, N., & De Giorgi, R. (1992). *Teoria della società*. Milano: Franco Angeli.

[89] Parsons, T., Bales, R.F. & Olds, J. (1955). *Family, Socialization and Interaction Process*. London: Routledge and Kegan Paul Ltd.

[90] Denzin, K. (1979). *Childhood Socialization*. San Francisco: Jossey-Bass.

[91] Alanen, L. (2001). Childhood as a Generational Condition, in Alanen, L. & Mayall B., *Conceptualising Child–Adult Relations*. London: Routledge/Falmer Press.

[92] Watzlawick, P., Bavelas, J. B., & Jackson, D. D. (2011). *Pragmatics of human communication: A study of interactional patterns, pathologies, and paradoxes*. WW: Norton & Company.

[93] Pagliaro, G., & Salvini, A. (2007). *Mente e psicoterapia*. Torino: *UTET.*

[94] Faccio, E., Iudici, A., Costa, N., & Belloni, E. (2014) Cyberbullying and interventions programs in school and clinical setting. In *Procedia-Social Behavioral Sciences*, vol. 122, p. 500-505.

[95] Iudici, A., & Faccio, E. (2014). What program works with bullying in school setting? Personal, social, and clinical implications of traditional and innovative intervention programs in *Procedia- Social Behavioral Sciences*, vol. 116, p. 4425-4429.

Chapter 7

INTERCULTURALITY AND SCHOOL: HISTORICAL REFERENCES, CONCEPTS AND METHODS OF INTERVENTION

1. INTRODUCTION

Some recent social changes, such as globalization, enlargement of the European Union, and the subsequent modification of the migration flows, have profoundly changed the way in which people interact. The major public and private actors involved in global governance of public health found the need for the integration and inclusion of people who were in a situation of disadvantage; these include the UN, WHO, and WTO. With the resolution "Health of Migrants" of WHO [1, 2, 3], the role of health was enshrined in promoting the process of the integration and social inclusion of third country nationals. Starting from the principle of the equality of rights, the United Nations [4, 5] proposed to organize society by using the resources in such a way as to ensure each individual had an equal chance to participate.

These macro changes have had a considerable impact on schools, which play a vital role in educating people in institutional interactions. The migration patterns of the last century have often led to situations in which people from very different cultural, social and school habits, from time to time, had to interact in the same territory. A necessary function of the school is to ensure that the interaction between people from different backgrounds is handled in a competent manner [6, 7, 8].

The ability to manage differences, however, cannot be delegated to the school, as it requires tools, methodologies and teaching methods very different from those with which the school has been supplied, having historically developed on the purely educational side. Besides, many of the actions that the school can put in place should be coordinated within a nationwide approach of the social-cultural country in which the school is located; otherwise, there is a great risk of fragmentation between what the schools produce and what the country wants. In addition, the integration policies, both institutional and within the school, must take into account some specific data from that country; for example, the migration flow, the historicity and the type of migration, and the country's ability to absorb this flow under the economic, social, and cultural profile [9].

It is necessary to study interventions not based on emergency situations, as these expose schools to continuous actions of adjustment, which make the work inconsistent and fragmented. The planning of activities, critical to any type of school, is rejected and troubled by urgent actions, creating the conditions for ineffective teaching and for the implementation of extemporaneous integration processes. Another requirement is to ensure that foreign students are treated not as a problem to be solved, but as a new scenario that must be managed by the same school organization. First, therefore, the school is required (with the mandate of the country) to choose its own way of tackling this phenomenon. This comes from the identification of an approach to cultural issues based on economic, social and cultural considerations, which must be explained on a general level and then shared by the micro-institutions (such as the school) [10].

2. Historical and Standard References

It is of particular interest, therefore, to observe the ways in which educational systems of different states and countries, and in different historical moments, have responded to the inclusion in their structures of students not belonging to the cultural reality of that context. For this purpose, it is useful to focus on the experiences of France, England, Germany and Italy regarding the interventions in education of the children of foreigners. From these experiences, we will highlight what approaches are used today in the face of cultural phenomena such as those described above.

2.1. The French Experience

With its ideals of liberty, equality and fraternity, the French educational institution sets up the practice of hospitality from two approaches: the assimilationist and the multicultural approaches.

Such approaches are inevitably affected by the historical conditions in which they are implemented. For example, the assimilationist approach was born in the post-colonial era (1950-1960), in which there was the peak of the process of decolonization [11]. The interest in favor of naturalization led to the recognition of French nationality to the children of foreigners born in France. This led to the political incorporation of immigrants and the fallout was a cultural and religious pluralism, which was new among the old European societies [12].

The legal instrument used was the principle of *ius soli*, according to which one who is born in the territory of a Member State is considered an original citizen, irrespective of the nationality of the parents. The impact of this approach was that people placed no value on their original cultural identity; what was important was what they aspired to, not where they came from. This had an impact even in school systems, being considered as an explanation of failure and the difficulty of integration, aspects related to social-economic boundaries, but not aspects of cultural differences. In fact, aspects such as learning difficulties and differences in how they perceived school or their relationships with teachers and classmates were not considered.

Starting from the 1960s, the realization dawned that considering an immigrant born in France as a French citizen was not in itself sufficient to produce integration [13].

The focus then shifted to the problems associated with cultural differences, those of creating a multicultural approach. The first difficulty encountered related to language difficulties, then considered a real "handicap". In order to reduce these difficulties, targeted experimental interventions were organized, which took the form of remedial classes for the children of foreigners residing in France, and of initiation classes. Then they proceeded by identifying the causes that prevented the full integration of immigrant children and, after having dealt with language issues, other factors were considered, which were mainly psychological - for example, the culture shock inherent in the transition from one cultural system to another, the dissonance between the cultural tradition of the family of origin and the host community or the presence of real psychological disorders (trauma, personality disorders, etc.). In this approach, the attention and respect for other cultures is proportional to the difficulties encountered; in fact, cultural differences were seen as a problem to be overcome.

The result of these two approaches gave rise to special psycho-pedagogical interventions and itineraries for foreign students, initially based on social-economic issues, then on ethnic-cultural aspects. Interventions were organized toward the so-called "*nouveaux arrivants*", which took place through *Classes d'initiation* and *Cours de Rattrapage Integré*, with the function, respectively, of courses for beginners to the French language and remedial courses and support for children with language difficulties [14].

Depending on the age and number, newcomers could be incorporated in the class *pré-professionnelle de niveau* or in *classes d'adaptation*, in which language support was provided, including, when possible, the opportunity to maintain ties with the language of origin. Then they created language and culture of origin courses for foreign students and, since 1980, became active projects of *zones d'education prioritaire*, with the aim of preventing situations of deviance and social discomfort [15]. Educational interventions promoted in France can therefore be described as pedagogical interventions for foreigners [16].

2.2. The English Experience

In this case some specific historical conditions facilitate the use of specific intervention policies. Migration flows are interwoven with the rules implemented with regard to the historical social needs [17]. The first significant intervention was the *Nationality Act* of 1948, which made it possible for all citizens of the Commonwealth[1], including therefore the inhabitants of the former colonies, to move freely within the borders of the empire with the status of British citizens [18].

After this document was published the first phase of migration began, which involved those who began with the intention to leave the country temporarily, usually without families, to earn enough money to reinvest once returning home. However, the diversion of the funds of the former colonies to the Sovereign State made it impossible for the creation of local industries and

[1] The Commonwealth of Nations, commonly known as the Commonwealth (also, the British Commonwealth), is an intergovernmental organization of 54 member states that were mostly territories of the former British Empire. They all consider Great Britain the leading country but they are all independent.

new jobs, thus creating conditions of poverty and marginalization among many immigrants.

A second phase of migration was represented by unmarried workers beginning to settle permanently in the host country [19]. The Commonwealth Act of 1962 defined the restrictive measures and drastically reduced the chances of immigration from countries of the Commonwealth [20]. A third phase of migration was that of the so-called migration chains, involving whole families, made up of women and children, from which arose the need for welfare programs. A relapse of the third phase was to create places in the city inhabited mainly by foreigners. Therefore, neighborhoods flourished inhabited mainly by communities which sought to reproduce the social structure of the area of origin [21].

If in the first two phases mentioned above one can recognize an assimilationist model, in order to maintain identification with the host environment, in the later stages the need to cope in different ways with the significant presence of different cultural systems increased. They therefore applied a multicultural approach to the problem, with the intention to produce integration from respect for different cultures. In this regard, the Race Relations Act was issued to eliminate racial discrimination in the workplace, in education and in public services [22, 23].

Specific rules were introduced to punish the specific conduct of social discrimination. In pedagogical terms, this gave rise, as in France, to efforts to overcome the deficit of immigrants, through the respect of their culture. Specificity of the Anglo-Saxon context was the initiatives against cultural discrimination, especially racism. In order to monitor the situation of minorities in school, an "ad hoc" committee was established in 1985, the *Committee of Inquiry into the Education of Children from Ethnic Minority Groups*, which produced a document, the Swann Report [24]. In this report the duties of education in a multicultural society were explained, in which "diversity" is recognized as a fundamental value and as an instrument of cohesion of the nation [25]. In addition, the need for a shift from an assimilationist approach to a pluralistic and multicultural one was considered, with all its inherent difficulties, such as language, religion, school integration.

From these requirements, two other legislative initiatives have helped to define the role of the school, the *Education Reform Act* of 1988 and the *Children Act* of 1989. The first document aimed to raise educational standards and the standardization of the training proposal, while the second enjoined all schools to ensure that every student of any race was afforded the necessary care, in terms of cultural, linguistic or materials, in school as at home [26].

In reference to the historic elements of legislation mentioned above, four different approaches that have alternated over the past fifty years can be found in the English school system.

The initial approach can certainly be defined as assimilationist, as it tended to create the conditions to assimilate foreign culture in English. At school level, the priority initiatives were guided by the objective of reducing the socio-cultural limitations of foreign students and for this reason were defined as "compensatory education". In operational terms, this meant teaching the language, history, traditions and values of Great Britain, so that foreigners could fit into the society of the “whites” in a situation of minimized conflict.

A second approach was the multicultural one, whose essential characteristics are identified in an attempt to differentiate between the various cultures of origin, promoting mutual respect. During this approach, many enhancement measures of the different communities in the area grew with the intention of triggering a constructive dialogue between the majority group and the minority. Even if the premises remained anchored to the idea of the “deficits” of the foreign entity, nevertheless, this approach was also open to the involvement of foreign students, with a view of pluralism.

Subsequently, to this day, it outlines an approach defined as intercultural education, but with few practical acts to distinguish the approach as multicultural.

2.3. The German Experience

Unlike the French and Anglo-Saxon context, the historical conditions of Germany created other realities and other types of intervention. The reasons for emigration in Germany were mainly two: the first, dating back to the late ’60s, was about the demand for labor in the industrial system, and the second was about the integration processes emerging after the fall of the Berlin Wall [27]. The first requirement produced the conception of immigrant guest workers, and was mainly represented by individuals without families, determined to earn enough money to invest in their country of origin [28]. The opening of the borders quickly increased the presence of these workers, inducing policies that would also allow the acceptance of their families. Neighborhoods were created with a high concentration of foreigners, where they lived “at a distance” with respect to the natives, tending to form homogeneous groups, sometimes in rivalry with other immigrant groups. This led to the abandonment of those places by the Germans [29].

Starting from this situation, educational initiatives of multiculturalism were produced in the '70s, called *Ausländerpädagogik*, educational activities for foreigners [30]. These activities assumed the differentiation of cultures, in order to create conditions of mutual respect. They organized pedagogical paths parallel to the normal ones, favoring the emergence of many special schools and the creation of special reception classes. Even in this case, the logic was kind of compensatory; immigrant students were considered Germans with linguistic and cultural gaps.

These strategies therefore concerned on one hand assimilation and integration into German society, and on the other the maintenance of their cultural identity. Subsequently, with the consolidation of migration and the presence of so-called second generation, initiation strategies of intercultural education were taken, aiming to create situations of social integration, although the main purpose remained to reduce the disadvantages in school.

2.4. The Italian Experience

The situation in Italy is unusual, since a country historically of emigration has become a country of immigration. Starting from the end of the 19th century, Italian citizens emigrated in a non-continuous flow to the United States of America and other European countries, succeeded by a period in which, at the end of the '70s, Italy was quickly hit by fast-growing migration flows and had to deal with the problem of the integration of foreigners, a completely new problem. In the early '80s the debate began, within the government, about the "stay of the non-EU citizen" and in 1986 the first Italian immigration law (Law No. 943 of 30/12/86) was issued, which focuses on the rules of placement and the treatment of foreign workers and immigrants against illegal immigration [31]. Unfortunately, this law proved ineffective with respect to the goals set forth and then it became necessary to produce a new piece of legislation, the so-called "Martelli law", l. no. 39 of 28.02.90, which, beyond the limits of the l. no. 943/1986, did not treat the foreigner only as an employee, but also introduced important provisions relating to the residence and outlined various interventions against the migrant [32]. This law, although more detailed than the previous one, was unable to cope with the migration. In 1998 another law was enacted, more systematic than the previous Law no. 40 of 6th March 1998 ("Rules and regulations on the immigration status of aliens"). Its purpose was to manage migration flows, to prevent and combat illegal immigration and to regulate social integration, dealing with the residence permit, family, children and civil rights. This law marks the boundary from the stage of the "discovery" of immigrants to the legislative definition of their rights, albeit chaotic and inaccurate, i.e. in the absence of a proper immigration policy.

The opening phase is characterized by the development and adoption of a policy of flows and inclusion (integration), providing at least economic and social rights [33]. The idea was to promote active migration policies, leaning toward social innovation projects.

Regarding the relationship between the educational system and foreign students, the management started with a perspective of intercultural education, formalized by some ministerial circulars. The first was the Ministerial Circular no. 301/1989, before the "Martelli" law, whereby they assumed the burden of summarizing the regulatory framework, national and international, regarding migrants' rights, and educational legislation that would make possible the acquisition of operational resources and the implementation of flexible modes of intervention. The aim was to promote their participation in the global activities of the class - for example, through initiatives of updating teachers and linguistic-cultural training. The measure refers to the duty of the school to consider the characteristics of a multicultural society and thus to promote educational activities aimed at enhancing the peculiarities of the different ethnic groups.

With the next circular, the Ministerial Circular no. 205/1990, entitled "*Compulsory education and foreign students*", some more innovative provisions were introduced, interventions to be carried out even in the absence of foreign students, in order to promote diversity and to promote a constructive coexistence [32].

In April of '92 the "*Intercultural Dialogue Week*" was promoted and on the 28th of the same month the CNPI (National Council of Public Education) produced a new circular. Ministerial Circular no. 122/1992 stated that intercultural education should be an educational perspective for all students and that the question of the presence of foreign and non-EU students makes clear the need for intercultural education. The Ministerial Circular no. 73/1994 entitled "*Intercultural dialogue and democratic society: the effort of the school*" is also significant, in which the government tried to increase awareness of teacher training with an intercultural perspective and to promote the construction of a "network culture" among all stakeholders [33]. This series of circulars, while directing the action in accordance with the purposes of social integration, carried with it the limitation that it did not represent a legislative apparatus capable of triggering structural changes to the social requirements coming forth [34]. The effect was to intervene based on emergencies, reducing the strength of the medium- and long-term measures. It is important to emphasize, however, that the actual landing point concerns the concept of intercultural education as directed both to foreign varieties, therefore not being reducible only to the former. In this sense, intercultural approaches begin to be seen as an interactive process between different cultures.

3. Approaches and Models

Also as a result of the above-mentioned experiences, we report below the approaches implemented toward social and cultural diversity. According to Gimenez [35], these approaches can be classified into exclusion and inclusion models. The differences are not always obvious, because the interventions were affected by different socio-political conditions and in many cases, the same approaches have overlapped one another, but it can be useful to distinguish the main characteristics. The classification below stands as an example of the main characteristic features of the types of approach.

3.1. Exclusion Model

The purpose of this approach is to keep pure and untainted the distinctive values of the culture of origin. The result is to prevent any form of contact between different cultural worlds, as well as the foreclosure of all occasions of social interaction. In this model it is possible to recognize three intervention policies: those discriminatory laws and practices based on industry; segregationist practices of those employing spatial exclusion (residential ghettos or delimitation of public spaces) and institutional (school segregation or health), those rounds based on elimination of the practices, both cultural (ethnocide and cultural fundamentalism) and physical (genocide and ethnic cleansing). In extreme cases, there is the possibility that different cultural identities co-exist in the same territory, but the important thing is that members of the host community respect the distances. This model denies foreigners the possibility of adopting the customs and traditions of the host culture [36].

3.2. Inclusion Model

The models of inclusion differ from those of exclusion by trying to give an answer of "integration" with respect to the issues of unity and social and cultural diversity. With this in mind, we try to relate the dominant culture with those of the minority [35]. Inscribed in this model are the so-called policy of homogenization (assimilation) and acceptance of cultural diversity.

3.2.1. The Monoculture or Homogenization Prospective

This approach has been applied through practices of cultural fusion, as in the case of Australia, Canada and the United States (in this context called a melting pot or salad bowl), and practices of assimilation, identified in France and England, from the mid-1940s until the 1980s. The basic idea of assimilationist policies is that minority cultural groups in the area should be integrated into the majority through a unilateral process of cultural absorption. In these practices the strangers, the representatives of a national minority, should then renounce their characteristics and their cultural identity and adopt without reservation the schemes and cultural behavior of the majority [37].

The denial and rejection of the culture of "foreigner" has not been without consequences; in fact, in many countries this has led to a strengthening of the positions against cultural minorities. In order to preserve their values of belonging, the latter have not only agreed to acquire the dominant culture as their own, but very often they are placed with respect to them in terms of contrast, in some cases through demonstrations of violence.

One of the most used legal terms is that of jus soli, meaning that anyone born within the borders of the state automatically becomes a citizen in all respects. In this way, the states facilitate and promote the development of citizenship. In short, the assimilation of a cultural group is based "on the approval of the other, whose specificities are concealed or denied as it is considered crucial the dominant cultural model, in which the alien must conform, with no space for possible mediation or negotiation" [38].

From an educational level, this approach means that there is a tendency to consider the teaching proposal as universal, the purpose of which is linguistic and cultural homogeneity, ignoring and not considering the presence of cultural differences [39]. The assumption of a mono-cultural perspective is to convey a unique system of social, cultural and economic references. The monocultural school assumes the existence of a given reality *a priori* from which the school acts to promote the integration and acceptance of "different" pupils. Reception and integration activities first try to overcome the disadvantage and/or the difference between the two types of students, and, on the other side, attest the existence of a diversity that distinguishes some from others.

3.2.2. The Multicultural and Pluricultural or the Acceptance Prospective

The cultural diversity policies are implemented in accordance with what can be termed as a "paradigm" of cultural pluralism, based on two *fundamental rights*, the *equality of rights* and the right to difference. From these rights are initially generated practices of multiculturalism but then, starting from an analysis of the critical points of the latter, those of interculturalism.

The multiculturalist's perspective is represented by those policies aimed at recognizing, protecting and ensuring the various cultural differences that exist in a particular country [40]. The practices that arise from this perspective focus on different areas, that of the right (with "*ad hoc*" assurance standards), religious, social services (specific measures of protection and assistance) and education (help in overcoming difficulties). The aim is to promote the acceptance of cultural diversity by welcoming people. In many cases this means organizing actions against the difficulties that foreign citizens, considered guests, meet by relating to the host culture. It is easy, often, to enter into a stereotyping and pathologizing process in which the difficulties of foreign students are translated into "psychological distress" (isolation stress) or "sociological marginality" (eradication stress) or "manifestation of psychopathology" (migratory trauma) [39]. The parameter from which to support the above is the "cultural norm" that inspired the host country.

The multiculturalist's practices, however, can lead to a kind of paradox, because the coexistence of different cultural worlds clearly precludes the ability to make viable a genuinely pluralist community. The ideological commitment to respecting cultural diversity and some folklore drifts have led to the inability to effectively promote social cohesion and cultural integration [35]. Another critical aspect is the implicit belief that culture is a static phenomenon and that defending this culture means not changing it. This concept has the effect of polarizing differences, though guided by the desire to preserve their existence. Despite these critical aspects, various initiatives have been signaled around the world to expand the cultural otherness, such as the Anglo-Saxon anti-racist movements of the '70s. Placing themselves in the defense of cultural diversity, these movements have attempted to counteract the dynamics through which racism originates and have promoted awareness of instances of racial discrimination in institutional, political, social, cultural, sporting and artistic contexts.

In education, this has resulted in action on two fronts: 1) socio-political, which traces the origin of racial differences in physical properties not as being cultural, but due to the imbalance in the distribution of power; 2) education, which analyzes the conflicts and possible solutions of the same, against the right of individuals to be able to develop to their full potential. This approach shifts the focus from those minority groups to the majority of the dominant culture, examining the rules of origin and the putting into practice of racist ideology. Overall, this setting hypostasizes the existence of "cultures" as static and irreducible to each other [41, 42].

3.2.3. The Intercultural Prospective

Among the inclusion models, this setting turns out to be the most recent, also, in relation to how this model managed to overcome some of the previous limitations. The conceptual references concerning the multicultural approach described above are therefore summarized in three aspects: understanding culture as if it were a "thing" that belongs to the individual or to the community and able to identify them uniquely. The second aspect concerns the assignment of a unique cultural identity of a community, from which descend personality traits peculiar to the individual belonging to that group ("the Romani are...", "Italians behave..."). Thirdly, it is believed that cultures have defined perimeters different from each other that we can clearly differentiate [43]. As you can see, the term culture is materialized and considered a fact.

The term establishes a basic property of a social group, identified as homogeneous inside and separated from other groups. It follows the idea that human societies take the form of an entity ideally closed, with attributes and permanent characteristics. In this case, the emphasis "is placed on elements within the group (its identity, its roots, its tradition) rather than on its placement in a wider system of relations. The boundaries are (ideally) waterproof and carefully supervised, hence the concern for the purity of tradition, seen as a "thing" to be protected against infection by isolating and protecting it from mingling with the outside world" [44]. These concepts produce two very critical consequences: first, stereotyped groups, Russians and Scots, Western and Eastern people, Christians and Muslims, as if they were in reality precisely distinct and distinguishable, with the same criterion of entomological classification or botanical taxonomy. Secondly, there is the so-called *ethnocentrism*, not being able to conceive, see, appreciate or recognize how positive are the multiple affiliations, areas of exchange and hybridization (perhaps inevitable) between different communities, as in the case of those persons or of those realities that can be identified neither in the native culture, nor in the "adoptive", and as Baumann says [45], are found to be "suspended between two cultures".

From the intercultural viewpoint the term culture is not reified, objectified, or considered statically, but it evokes a dynamic and procedural reality, although social workers and schools often confuse it with the multicultural approach.

Culture can be described as a device for the mediation of human experience [46], as a set of resources available to the action of individuals and social groups [47] or as a shared narrative, contested and negotiated among the various social actors [48]. In any case, we are referring to it as a particular "form" socially and historically situated, able to organize the experience and relationships of both individuals and social groups. UNESCO defines intercultural practice thus: *"who says intercultural, necessarily says, starting from the prefix "inter", interaction, exchange, openness, reciprocity, objective solidarity. It also says "culture": acknowledging the values, the ways of life, the symbolical representations to which human beings, individuals or societies relate to in their interaction with the others, and in understanding the world, recognizing their importance and the interactions which simultaneously interfere with the multiple registers of the same culture but also of different cultures."* [49].

Interculturalism emphasizes the understanding, care, promotion and regulation of socio-cultural relations and their consequences. Such conceptions (such as mediation systems, system resources for action, such as polyphonic narration) intersect with regard not to considering culture as a "monolith", a "thing" or a "phenotypic" property that defines the identity of a social group, but in defining human societies as open relational systems whose stories are constantly interconnected [46], which is the interweaving of the plots of these stories to form the identity of these groups of people. An example of an open relational system is the school, which is understood as a space of culture building, an area of active and shared research, only "cross-cultural" because it does not belong to one culture or another; it is generated by interaction between the participating parties [50, 51, 52]. The school thus becomes the context of the exchange, even between different cultural experiences, which can form new meanings and relational formulas, stamped by the restriction of stereotypes and ethnocentric[2] attitudes that often "live" common sense.

In this sense, cultural interaction becomes a fundamental process in the education system, applicable in every situation and in every part of the socialization of the land. Creating a school cross-cultural understanding as a space for the production of a shared culture involves abandoning the label of "foreign" and "Italian" and "disabled" or "inconvenient", to put the focus of each intervention on the pupil, understood as the role of student and citizen [54, 55]. In this sense, rather than focusing on cultural differences, it is to induce adherence to a social role in the organization of the country, both for the so-called foreigners, and for the so-called natives.

Gimenez [35] talks about the *principle of citizenship*, which implies the full recognition and the constant pursuit of substantive equality of rights, responsibilities, and opportunities. This is a role with respect to which belonging culture or expressed skills are no longer the focus of interventions [51, 56, 57]. The primary objective of intercultural interventions is therefore to lay the foundations for co-constructing different ratios, where differences do not represent a critical point, but an opportunity. Consequently, the identity is a construct that outlines a process of exchange that is created in the interaction with others, historically defined and permanently changing [58].

4. Method Indications to Promoting Health

Taking into account what has been said, some methodological indications are now offered for interventions in school from a perspective of health promotion regarding how cultural issues have been dealt with under the scientific perspective.

4.1. From Culture as an Entity to Culture as a Process

According to a reified view of culture, social groups present themselves as internally homogeneous and externally separated by insurmountable

---

[2] The term ethnocentrism is described as "a sense of superiority of the ways of acting and thinking over those characteristic of other societies and ethnic groups, a source of bias in judging the behavior of others". [53]

boundaries, fixed and permanent. This concept generates a system of cultural plurality, inside which takes shape multiculturalism as a "mosaic" pattern that provides for the coexistence, more or less peaceful, of different groups in which mixtures are not designed, but in which each maintains its own traditional identity. In school, this translates into trying to respect the cultural differences from the geographical places of origin. It is as if we were to respect the personal and cultural understanding of, for example, teaching lessons to a child from China and one from Colombia, as if those differences were ontologically given.

Otherwise, redefining culture as an exchange process that occurs in the interaction between different positions, the aim is to give a new meaning to the events. In this sense, the starting positions give rise to a shared vision, new, not previously existing, whose paternity is both. Consequently, the interculture coincides with the process of the same codetermination and the differences are the tool to come to a new position, of both.

The promotion of culture as a process leaves open spaces of exchanges and negotiations, able to generate new relationships. This does not exclude the differences between the positions; it leads to a focus on how to inter-operate those positions. The Chinese and Colombian students' viewpoint in Italy, for example, can contribute to experiencing lessons in a new way, even in relation to what the Italian school organization asks of that role.

4.2. From a Moral to a Projectual Viewpoint

Frequently, responsible teachers and operators dwell on the cultural habits of the children present at school and organize various activities (such as research and exhibitions) aimed at the moral respect of individual geography and culture.

In other situations, instead, teachers want foreign students and their families to adapt to the patterns and values of the host territory.

In both cases, the sense of respect becomes the fundamental objective for which to strive. The school-based intervention in respect of cultural differences is this way permeated by value judgments and moral claims. This has at least three consequences: first, considering culture as an objective entity, then believing that the ultimate goal is to respect the values of others and, thirdly, which every teacher can move in a non-shareable way because the values are subjective connotations.

From a cross-cultural perspective, respect for differences, dictated from a certain geographical origin, is not the goal for which to strive in moral terms, but the contribution from which students start to live together as the establishment or the role of the student requires. In methodological terms, this can be confused with the objectives of the intervention strategies and can occur exactly when you decide to intervene from a moral perspective, whereby every teacher is entitled to intervene in a personal way and not through a shared project. Only through a project led by clear objectives can the various operators bring together their efforts of intervention in a precise way, without any loss of economic or temporal drifts and personalistic attitudes. The implementation of practices based on personal goals is, in fact, highly detrimental to the effectiveness of cross-cultural projects, implicit rather than explicit, and shared, so that each operator can strive for the same success.

4.3. From the Foreign Stereotype to the Role of Student

Monocultural and multicultural approaches reify the concept of culture, considering some objective characteristics of people. The fallout is found in the context of everyday interpersonal relationships, which are filtered and interpreted according to some cultural stereotypes. For example, the concepts of "alien", "immigrant", and "second-generation foreign" imply *a priori* definition of the individual, based on cultural dogmas, with two consequences: 1) the triggering of a fictional relationship, based on criteria external to what would happen between people; 2) the distancing of oneself from what each institution requires, or not taking into consideration the role of the student. Acting toward others based on stereotypes means relating to a mysterious entity, formed by a supposed ontological conception of the other, at the expense of being able to act together to pursue shared objectives.

This type of injury may derive even from feelings and desires of integration, as we have seen in the cultural approach. However, in fact, if we relate to each other as "different", we are likely to build a relationship based on the difference, or even on opposition, whether we do this with noble intent, or through a preliminary mode. In school, thinking in terms of "role" means considering the resources of the individual in relation to their presence in the classroom and this is independent from criteria relating to the provenance or the criteria values.

It is therefore considered that the person is able to construct his/her own knowledge from his/her own actions and by placing these actions in relation to an institutional context, which requires students to interact with a view to the development of citizenship skills.

4.4. From the Student as a Passive Recipient to the Student as Intercultural Process Protagonist

Inside an intercultural view, the criterion of geographical origin/cultural habits is not a problem, but one of the contributions available with which to exercise one's role. This is especially true in light of the way in which the educational institution requires students to learn, or in the educational activities of the group. The institutional reference, as we have seen, is the role of the student, which has as its objective the development of citizenship skills, where the notional element is only one of the elements taken into account. In relation to this objective there is the need to break free from cultural and linguistic practices of indoctrination, enabling the full involvement of those who express themselves in ways they find useful. Consistent with this, we can move away from the idea of a passive student oriented to conform to what is suggested, to the idea of a student who makes his/her own contribution, even culturally, but not specifically. In this sense, the class group is home to ideas, concepts and different meanings as well as the ability to generate "new realities". The advantage of this is that you can take the opportunity to generate the "Knowing" from multiple resources, which are interchangeable and can lead to different concepts, each of which may be appropriate in certain situations and less relevant for others. The school and the community can therefore accommodate the comparison between those ideas, and thus produce an internal change as a function of changing social and cultural needs. The *sine qua non* of this process is to facilitate the full expression of the students, by taking an active role, and to encourage the development of skills relying on their direct experience.

REFERENCES

[1] World Health Organization (2008). *Health Of Migrants.* Sixty-First World Health Assembly. Geneva: WHO.

[2] Commission of the European Communities (2008). *Green Paper. Migration & mobility: challenges and opportunities for EU education systems*. Brussels: http://eurlex.europa.eu/.

[3] Council of Europe (2008). *White Paper on Intercultural Dialogue. Living Together s Equals in Dignity*, Strasburg: www.coe.int/dialogue

[4] World Health Organization (2006). Regional Office for Europe's Health Evidence Network (HEN). *What is the evidence on effectiveness of empowerment to improve health?* Geneva: World Health Organization.

[5] World Health Organization (2007). *Schools for Health, Education and Development: A Call for Action.* Geneva: World Health Organization.

[6] Unesco (1960). *Convention against Discrimination in Education, Articles: 1, 3 and 4.* Paris: Unesco.

[7] Stenou, K. (2007). L'*Unesco et la question de la diversité culturelle 1946-2007: Bilan et stratégies*, in *série diversité culturelle n° 3*, (ed). Paris: Unesco.

[8] Ferri, D. (2005). EU Partecipation in the Unesco Convention on the Protection and Promotion of the Diversity of Cultural Expressions: Some Constitutional Remarks, *European Diversity and Autonomy Papers – EDAP*, at www.eurac.edu/edap

[9] Finnemore, M. (1993). International organizations as teachers of norms: The United Nations Educational, Scientific, and Cultural Organization and science policy. *International Organization*, 47(4), p. 565-597.

[10] Sekhar, A., & Steinkamp, A. (2010). *Mapping Cultural Diversity: Good Practices from around the Globe. A Contribution to the Debate on the Implementation of the UNESCO Convention on the Protection and Promotion of the Diversity of Cultural Expressions*: a Project of the U40-programme "Cultural Diversity 2030". German Commission for UNESCO & Asia-Europe Foundation. Germany: Rheinbreitbach.

[11] Kastoryano, R. (1996). *La France, l'Allemagne et leurs immigrés: Négocier l'identité* [*France, Germany and their immigrants: Negotiating identity*]. Paris: Armand Colin.

[12] Caputo, M. (1999). Pedagogia nazionale e universalismo laico: le pratiche interculturali nella scuola francese. In Damiano, E. (A cura di), *La sala degli specchi. Pratiche scolastiche di Educazione interculturale in Europa* (p. 56-115). Milano: Franco Angeli.

[13] Noiriel, G. (1996). *The French melting pot: Immigration, citizenship and national identity*. Minneapolis: University of Minnesota Press.

[14] Lazaridis, M. (2001). La scolarisation des enfants de migrants: entre intégration républicaine et mesures spécifiques. Paris: *Ville-Ecole-Intégration Enjeux*, n. 125, p. 198-208.

[15] Bénabou, R., Kramarz, F., Prost, C. (2004). Zones d'éducation prioritaire: quels moyens pour quels résultats? Une évaluation sur la période 1982-1992. *Économie et Statistique* (380), p. 3-29.
[16] Brubaker, R. (2001). The Return of Assimilation? Changing Perspectives on Immigration and Its Sequels in France Germany and the United States. *Ethnic and Racial Studies*, 24 (4), p. 531-548.
[17] Favell, Adrian (1997) Citizenship and immigration: pathologies of a progressive philosophy, in: *New Community*, 23(2), p. 173-195.
[18] Giromini, M. (1999). Il conflitto organizzato: educazione interculturale e antirazzista in Gran Bretagna. In E. Damiano (A cura di), *La sala degli specchi. Pratiche scolastiche di Educazione interculturale in Europa*. Milano: Franco Angeli.
[19] Goel, U. (1998). *Citizenship and Identity among Second Generation South Asians in Western European Countries.* MA dissertation. School of Oriental and African Studies, University of London. Available at www.urmila.de/UDG/Biblio/Citizenship.pdf (accessed on 14.04.2013.
[20] Hepple, B.A. (1968). Commonwealth Immigrants Act. *The Modern Law Review*. vol. 31, (4), p. 424-428.
[21] Jacobson, J. (1997). Perceptions of Britishness, in *Nations and Nationalism*, 3(2), p. 181-199).
[22] McCrudden, C. (1985) Changing Notions of Discrimination, in Stephen Guest & Alan Milne, *Equality and discrimination: essays in freedom and justice* 83, 84.
[23] Hepple, B. (1992). Have Twenty-five Years of the Race Relations Act in Britain Been a Failure?, in Hepple, B., & Szyszczak, E., *Discrimination: the Limits of Law*. London: Mansell.
[24] Swann, L. (1985). *Education For All: The Report of the Inquiry into the Education of Children from Ethnic Minority Groups*. London: HMSO.
[25] Cohen, R. (1995). Fuzzy frontiers of identity: the British case. *Social Identities*, 1(1), p. 35-62.
[26] Neave, G. (1988). On the cultivation of quality, efficiency, and enterprise: An overview of recent trends in higher education in Western Europe, 1986–1988. *European Journal of Education* 23 (1/2), p. 7-23.
[27] Mehrländer, U., Ascheberg, C., & Ueltzhöffer, J. (1996), *Repräsentativuntersuchung '95. Situation der ausländischen Arbeitnehmer und ihrer Familienangehörigen in der Bundesrepublik Deutschland.* Bundesministerium für Arbeit und Sozialordnung, Bonn.

[28] Kurthen, H. (1995). Germany at the crossroads: national identity and the challenges of immigration. *International Migration Review*, 29 (4), p. 914-938.

[29] Bombardelli, O. (1999). Accogliere differenziando. Educazione interculturale ed educazione politica nelle scuole della Germania federale. In Damiano, E. (A cura di), *La sala degli specchi. Pratiche di Educazione interculturale in Europa*. Milano: Franco Angeli.

[30] Diehm, I., & Radtke, F.O. (1999). *Erziehung und Migration.* Stuttgart. Köln: Kohlhammer

[31] Todeschini, P., Caputo, M., & Cipollari, G. (1999). Dall'alto e dal basso. Il "caso" italiano. In E. Damiano (A cura di), *La sala degli specchi. Pratiche scolastiche di educazione interculturale in Europa* (p. 282-362). Milano: Franco Angeli.

[32] Zincone, G. (1995). Immigration Policies in Italy. In Heckmann, F. & Bosswick, W. (eds.), *Migration policies. A comparative perspective*, Forum Migration no. 1, second edition, Stuttgart: Enke.

[33] Caponio, T. (2008). Immigration research in Italy: A European comparative Perspective. *The Sociological Quarterly*, 49, p. 445-464.

[34] Ongini, V., (2001). *Lo scaffale multiculturale*. Milano: Mondadori.

[35] Giménez, C. (2008). Interculturalismo. In G. Mantovani (A cura di), Intercultura *e mediazione. Teorie ed esperienze* (p. 149-169). Roma: Carocci.

[36] Di Marco, G., Hichy, Z., & Sapienza, I. (2012). Effetti dell'empatia sull'adozione delle strategie di acculturazione nei confronti degli immigrati albanesi. *Annali della facoltà di Scienze della formazione.* Università degli studi di Catania, p. 127-139.

[37] Martiniello, M. (2000). Gestire la diversità culturale e identitaria. *Rivista online: Il Mulino* (5), p. 881-889. DOI: 10.1402/997.

[38] Mongelli, A. (2008). L'intercultura: dalla teoria alle pratiche. In Boffo, V. & Torlone, F. (A cura di), *L'inclusione sociale e il dialogo interculturale nei contesti europei. Strumenti per l'educazione, la formazione e l'accesso al lavoro* (p. 60-75). Firenze: Firenze University Press.

[39] Damiano, E. (1999). (A cura di) *La sala degli specchi. Pratiche scolastiche di Educazione interculturale in Europa.* Milano: Franco Angeli.

[40] Kymlicka, W. (1999). *La cittadinanza multiculturale*. Bologna: Il Mulino.

[41] Krystyna, M., & Bleszynska, A. (2008). Constructing intercultural education. *Intercultural Education*, 19, (p. 537-545).
[42] Aime, M. (2004). *Eccessi di culture*. Torino: Einaudi.
[43] Mantovani, G. (2008). Intercultura: la differenza in casa. In G. Mantovani, *Intercultura e mediazione. Teorie ed esperienze* (p. 17-31). Roma: Carocci Editore.
[44] Mantovani, G. (2006). Il difficile riconoscimento delle differenze. La necessità di una scelta tra due concezioni incompatibili di cultura. *Psicologia Sociale* (2), 223-232.
[45] Baumann, G. (1996). *Contesting culture. Discourses of identity in multi-ethnic London*. Cambridge: Cambridge University Press.
[46] Cole, M. (1996). *Cultural psychology. A once and future discipline*. Cambridge: Harvard Huniversity Press.
[47] Mantovani, G. (2004). *Intercultura. È possibile evitare le guerre culturali?* Bologna: Il Mulino.
[48] Benhabib, S. (2002). *The claims of culture. Equality and diversity in the global era*. Princeton: Princeton University Press.
[49] Unesco (1980). *Introduction aux études interculturelles: esquisse d'un projet pour l'élucidation et la promotion de la communication entre les cultures*. Unesco, 1976-1980. Paris: Unesco.
[50] Lahdenperä, P. (2000). From monocultural to intercultural educational research, *Intercultural Education*, 11, p. 201-207.
[51] Coulby, D. (2006). Intercultural education: theory and practice. *Intercultural Education*, 17, p. 245-257.
[52] Culla, L., & Turchi G.P. (2005). *Stranieri e Droghe. Dalla cura del corpo alle pratiche discorsive nel sistema carcerario*. Roma: Armando Editore.
[53] Marrazzi, A. (1998). *Lo sguardo antropologico. Processi educativi e multiculturalismo*. Roma: Carocci.
[54] Iudici, A., De Aloe, S., Fornaro, G., Priori, M., & Strada, A. (2013). Countering the "career of disability": from clinical institutionalization to the creation of opportunities for biographical change. The intervention of the Service for Integration, Accompaniment and Orientation for students with disabilities of the Municipalities of Melzo and Liscate (Mi). In *Procedia - Social and Behavioral Sciences,* Elsevier Ltd, vol. 116, Pages 3271-3275.

[55] Iudici, A. (2014). Skills-Lab Project- Promoting the integration of diversity as a culture of participation. Community relief, economic, social, clinical and health in *Procedia- Social Behavioral Sciences*, Volume 116, Pages 3636-3640, Elsevier Ltd.

[56] Perry, L.B., & Southwell, L. (2011). Developing intercultural understanding and skills: models and approaches. *Intercultural Education*, 22, p. 453-466.

[57] Spitzberg, B.H. (2000). A Model of Intercultural Communication Competence. In Samovar, L.A. & Porter, R.E. *Intercultural Communication. A Reader* (p. 375-87). Belmont: Wadsworth Publishing.

[58] Berger, P., & Luckman, T. (1966). *The Social Construction of Reality: A Treatise its the Sociology of Knowledge*. Garden City, New York: Anchor Books.). Trad.it. Berger, P., Luckman, T. (1969). *La realtà come costruzione sociale.* Bologna: Il Mulino.

INDEX

C

D

E

F

G

H

I

J

L

M

N

O

P

Q

R

S

T

U

V

W

Y